Professional
Well-Being

Enhancing Wellness Among Psychiatrists, Psychologists, and Mental Health Clinicians

Professional Well-Being

Enhancing Wellness Among Psychiatrists, Psychologists, and Mental Health Clinicians

By
Grace W. Gengoux, Ph.D., BCBA-D
Sanno E. Zack, Ph.D.
Jennifer L. Derenne, M.D.
Athena Robinson, Ph.D.
Laura B. Dunn, M.D.
Laura Weiss Roberts, M.D., M.A.

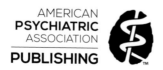

AMERICAN
PSYCHIATRIC
ASSOCIATION
PUBLISHING

If you wish to buy 50 or more copies of the same title, please go to www.appi.org/specialdiscounts for more information.

First Edition

Manufactured in the United States of America on acid-free paper
24 23 22 21 20   5 4 3 2 1

American Psychiatric Association Publishing
800 Maine Avenue SW
Suite 900
Washington, DC 20024-2812
www.appi.org

Library of Congress Cataloging-in-Publication Data
Names: Gengoux, Grace W., author. | American Psychiatric Association, issuing body.
Title: Professional well-being : enhancing wellness among psychiatrists, psychologists, and mental health clinicians / by Grace W. Gengoux, Sanno E. Zack, Jennifer L. Derenne, Athena Robinson, Laura B. Dunn, Laura Weiss Roberts.
Description: First edition. | Washington, D.C. : American Psychiatric Association Publishing, [2020] | Includes bibliographical references and index.
Identifiers: LCCN 2020001995 (print) | LCCN 2020001996 (ebook) | ISBN 9781615372294 (paperback) | ISBN 9781615373086 (ebook)
Subjects: MESH: Burnout, Professional | Psychology | Mental Health | Psychiatry | Self Care
Classification: LCC RC455 (print) | LCC RC455 (ebook) | NLM WM 62 | DDC 616.89—dc23
LC record available at https://lccn.loc.gov/2020001995
LC ebook record available at https://lccn.loc.gov/2020001996

British Library Cataloguing in Publication Data
A CIP record is available from the British Library.

To my family, for inspiring me to do work that matters.—G.W.G.

*To my DBT Team, who strive every day to make well-being their corner-
stone and without whom I could not thrive.*
Thank you for your generous hearts.
And to Ed, my forever partner in the work-life balance two-step.
With love.—S.E.Z.

*For all the wonderful colleagues, patients, and trainees who educate me
every day, and remind me to practice what I try to teach.—J.L.D.*

*For my esteemed colleagues and the clients we have been honored to
work alongside.*
And to Jeffrey, for your endless support.—A.R.

For Jim, always.—L.B.D.

*For my colleagues, professionals who give so much of themselves for the
benefit of others.—L.W.R.*

Contents

Part I
Well-Being and Wellness
An Emerging Imperative for the Health Professions

Part II
Well-Being and Positive Self-Care
Practical Approaches for Psychiatrists and Mental Health Professionals

About the Authors

Grace W. Gengoux, Ph.D., BCBA-D, is a Clinical Associate Professor in the Department of Psychiatry and Behavioral Sciences at the Stanford University School of Medicine in Stanford, California.

Sanno E. Zack, Ph.D., is a Clinical Associate Professor in the Department of Psychiatry and Behavioral Sciences at the Stanford University School of Medicine in Stanford, California.

Jennifer L. Derenne, M.D., is a Clinical Professor in the Department of Psychiatry and Behavioral Sciences at the Stanford University School of Medicine in Stanford, California.

Athena Robinson, Ph.D., is Chief Clinical Officer, Woebot Labs, Inc.

Laura B. Dunn, M.D., is a Professor in the Department of Psychiatry and Behavioral Sciences at the Stanford University School of Medicine in Stanford, California.

Laura Weiss Roberts, M.D., M.A., is Chairman and Katharine Dexter McCormick and Stanley McCormick Memorial Professor in the Department of Psychiatry and Behavioral Sciences at Stanford University School of Medicine; Chief of Psychiatry Service at the Stanford Hospital and Clinics, Stanford, California; and Editor-in-Chief, Books, at American Psychiatric Association Publishing in Washington, D.C.

Disclosure of Competing Interests

The following contributor to this book has indicated a financial interest in or other affiliation with a commercial supporter, a manufacturer of a commercial product, a provider of a commercial service, a nongovernmental organization, and /or a government agency, as listed below:

Laura Weiss Roberts, M.D., M.A., serves as the Chairman and Katharine Dexter McCormick and Stanley McCormick Memorial Professor in the Department of Psychiatry and Behavioral Sciences at the Stanford University School of Medicine. She owns Terra Nova Learning Systems (TNLS), a small company that develops science-based educational products.

Dr. Roberts has received federal funding for competitive, peer-reviewed research grants and competitive, peer-reviewed small business grants and contracts. The key stakeholders, such as Stanford University and the NIH, are fully aware of this arrangement and have given prior approval for this set of professional commitments. In addition, she often serves as a consultant for federally funded scientific projects with collaborators across the United States.

Dr. Roberts is the Editor-in-Chief, Books, at American Psychiatric Association Publishing. Funds associated with these duties are provided to Stanford University. Dr. Roberts does not receive direct funding from pharmaceutical companies for her work, and she is not on "Speakers' Bureaus" of any kind. She does give academic and public/community talks for which she receives honoraria.

Dr. Roberts has published books and receives royalties. These royalties represent a very small proportion of Dr. Roberts' overall income

The following contributors have indicated that they have no financial interests or other affiliations that represent or could appear to represent a competing interest with the contributions to this book:

Jennifer L. Derenne, M.D., Laura B. Dunn, M.D., Grace W. Gengoux, Ph.D., BCBA-D, Athena Robinson, Ph.D., and Sanno E. Zack, Ph.D.

Preface

Very early one morning as a second-year medical student, I went to the Coronary Care Unit at a university-affiliated hospital. I was hoping to find a patient willing to tell his story—of developing heart disease, of experiencing a cardiac event, of living with chronic heart failure—because I had a write-up due later that afternoon. On the whiteboard on the wall, a patient's initials were scrawled next to the letters "TCA OD."

Instead of finding that those initials belonged to a stranger admitted to the unit, I discovered, by accident, that they belonged to a friend. A classmate. A wonderful colleague who had attempted suicide with tricyclic antidepressants the night before. For confidentiality reasons, the clinical team planned on transferring him to another hospital, but they hadn't yet been able to stabilize him. I had arrived too early in the morning. He was still there. He saw me see him, and he read my concern. An understanding quickly passed between us.

I had another classmate, a brilliant guy who drank vodka each day, the bottle hidden in the gross anatomy laboratory, the telltale scent of vodka masked by the smell of cadavers. Another classmate's Crohn's disease wasn't diagnosed until he nearly bled to death from a ruptured ulcer. His doctor previously had said that his symptoms were stress related (probably "medical student syndrome"). Then, there is my own story. I had a baby during medical school. And, inevitably, I had complications, and—thankfully—salutary outcomes, both for my daughter and for myself.

The classmate with depression graduated with honors a few years later, as did the one with the vodka habit. The one with Crohn's left medicine altogether.

And I went on to become a psychiatrist. Caring for the physical and mental health of medical students, residents, and health care professionals has been an important part of my work each day since those formative experiences in medical school. It has been a great joy to engage clinically with my colleagues as well as to develop and oversee novel health programs for physicians, physicians-in-training, and other health professionals. Conducting research has been especially compelling and inspiring.

We are learning that clinicians do not need to be superhuman to be good doctors. Clinicians with an understanding of their own health needs may be more attuned and compassionate toward their patients, and clinicians with strong personal self-care habits may be more attentive to the preventive health and health-related behaviors of their patients. Clinicians who are mindful of their own vulnerability, resilience, and strength may be especially gifted in taking care of patients, living with a deep sense of purpose and using their experiences in the service of health professions.

Together, we are seeking to create a new culture and a new way of being. This new culture includes ways of being organized and ways of doing things that are supportive of the health and well-being of health professionals and the health and well-being of the patients and populations we serve. Creating this new culture, replete with new expectations of ourselves and one another, is not easy, but it is essential. The mental health professions are overwhelmed by the needs of patients throughout the world, as well as those of our colleagues and learners in the clinics, laboratories, classrooms, and communities that surround us. To do all that we can, we must endeavor to care for ourselves and to align our strengths with the work that we are called to do.

This book is the result of a close collaboration of several psychiatrist and psychologist colleagues in the Department of Psychiatry and Behavioral Sciences in the School of Medicine at Stanford University. Each of the collaborators has brought an important perspective and a wealth of expertise and experience working in the area of mental and physical health of clinicians and clinicians-in-training. I offer my gratitude to this wonderful collaborative team for our work together. On behalf of all of the coauthors, I also offer our heartfelt thanks and appreciation to Michelle Lau, who transformed this manuscript with her editing expertise, and to Lingfei Ni, Ann Tennier, Gabrielle Termuehlen, and Tenzin Tsungmey for their outstanding work in the development of this manuscript.

Laura Weiss Roberts, M.D., M.A.
Stanford, California
July 2019

PART I

Well-Being and Wellness

An Emerging Imperative for the Health Professions

CHAPTER 1

Healthy Clinicians, Healthy Patients

Mental health care, at its core, is about promoting the psychological health and overall well-being of patients. Decades of research and clinical practice have focused on the very important goal of developing and disseminating evidence-based practices for enhancing mental health for a wide range of patient populations. A growing recognition of the importance of self-care for psychiatrists and psychologists themselves is now emerging. This goal is important for the health of all mental health professionals and for the health of their patients.

Mental health professionals may struggle to implement their own self-care. The culture of medicine has historically valued the ideals of self-sacrifice and perfectionism. As a result, psychiatrists and psychologists frequently report feeling guilty or self-indulgent when they take the time and effort to enhance their own wellness and quality of life. Professionals with mental disorders, substance-related conditions, or behavioral problems, in particular, are exposed to distinct and difficult stresses.

Appropriate self-consideration is respectful of one's patients and oneself and essential for competent practice. To be effective, clinicians

---

must be energetic, connected to others, and knowledgeable about preventive health and self-care. The fields of psychiatry and psychology have much to contribute regarding wellness, even as psychiatrists and psychologists face unique threats to well-being while they help others to bear considerable trauma, distress, and suffering.

This book was written for psychiatrists, psychologists, and other mental health professionals who care for patients across a full range of practice settings. Information has been included that is applicable throughout the professional life span, including for students and trainees. For reasons of brevity and readability, the text focuses primarily on psychiatrists and psychologists. However, the intention is to be inclusive of all mental health professionals at any level of training. The motivation behind this book is to offer inspiration, support, and practical strategies that can be employed by psychiatrists, psychologists, mental health clinicians, and trainees to advance professional and personal well-being.

Defining Well-Being

A singular and immense challenge in the field of physician well-being relates to how well-being is defined. A recent systematic review by Brady et al. (2018) explored the conceptualization of physician well-being. The project examined more than 2,400 published works and identified 78 relevant studies published on the topic between 1989 and 2015. Only 14% of the relevant papers provided an explicit definition of physician wellness. Mention of mental and social aspects of well-being were included in more than half of the papers, but dimensions of physical and integrated well-being were mentioned in fewer than half of the papers. A trend toward a more integrated model of wellness that includes mental, social, and physical dimensions was revealed in an analysis that compared papers published during 1989–2009 versus 2010–2015.

Brady et al. (2018) raised the issue of the need for high-quality research predicated on conceptual clarity. Such clarity is currently lacking, and the authors argued that much good would come from a consensus definition for physician wellness:

> We conclude that only a holistic definition of physician wellness will adequately improve medical practice. Anything less will merely perpetuate the cultural, organizational, and policy contexts in which physicians are often expected to deny their own wellness in favor of providing consistently compassionate and competent patient care, a situation we find neither beneficent nor efficient. (Brady et al. 2018, p. 106)

As outlined in Table 1–1, getting appropriate rest and exercise, accessing psychosocial support or mentoring, and experiencing meaning and purpose are a few of the many diverse contributors to achieving well-being.

Well-Being and Patient Outcomes

One reason for emphasis on health professional wellness is the growing recognition that when psychologists and psychiatrists are healthier, their patients benefit too. Self-care is particularly important, given that doctors who take better care of themselves also appear to take better care of their patients. For instance, data from diverse aspects of medical care (mammography, influenza vaccination, blood pressure screening, colorectal cancer screening) indicate that physician self-care is correlated with better patient care (Frank et al. 2010, 2013).

A long history of overwork and self-sacrifice in the medical field is now being criticized as unhelpful and even detrimental or dangerous to both clinician and patient health. Factors directly linked to high levels of stress among psychiatrists and psychologists include a difficult combination of heavy caseloads, limited control over the work environment, long hours, and financial and organizational strains. The resulting burnout creates a new kind of public health crisis in which highly educated and experienced health care workers leave the profession, exacerbating problems of access to necessary care for patients. The health of psychiatrists and psychologists is seen as an important business practice for sustainable positive impact and an emerging imperative for large health care organizations. Importantly, wellness programs must be respectful, sensitive to diversity, and not just another form of enforcing unrealistic perfectionism (Baker 2003).

Historical Roots of Wellness for Physicians

Although wellness has become an increasingly popular construct in contemporary life, the concept of caring for the self has deep roots in ancient philosophy, including in the practices of Ayurveda as well as ancient Greek and traditional Chinese medicine. The emergence of such fields as osteopathy, homeopathy, naturopathy, and chiropractic in the nineteenth century further set the stage for modern medicine's increasing acknowledgment that mental and spiritual well-being support physical health. As the concept of taking care of wellness (as opposed to illness) became even more mainstream at the end of the twentieth century, businesses began to incorporate wellness programming into their

TABLE 1–1. Key drivers of physician wellness

Domain	Contributors to well-being	Detractors from well-being
Mental well-being	Job satisfaction	Emotional exhaustion
	Positive mood	Anxiety, depression
	Self-esteem	Low sense of accomplishment
Social well-being	Adaptation	Isolation and alienation
	Participation	Depersonalization
Physical well-being	Work-rest balance	Sleep problems and fatigue
	Exercise behaviors	Alcohol or tobacco use
Integrated well-being	Life satisfaction	

Source. Adapted from Brady et al. 2018.

employee benefits. Today, it is increasingly common to discuss issues of professional well-being across a wide range of disciplines.

In parallel with the growing focus on wellness in the general population, important historical movements in medicine paved the way for drastic change in thinking about the health of doctors themselves. The transition from seeing doctors as individuals with godlike powers to seeing doctors as human beings in need of support and caregiving has taken a long time and has been met with considerable resistance. Yet the mind-set change has had critical benefits for psychiatrists, psychologists, and patients alike.

Many of the barriers to acknowledging the importance of physician wellness have come from inside the field of medicine itself, driven by the sometimes fiercely held myth that to be a good doctor one must be superhuman. Aspects of medical training and practice reinforce this perfectionistic attitude, for instance, by creating training schedules that normalize unsafe sleep deprivation and medical licensure application questions about prior mental health treatment. Figure 1–1 depicts a striking reluctance to seek mental health care among American surgeons, attributed largely to fears about potential medical licensure repercussions (Shanafelt et al. 2011).

Trainees and practicing physicians may even neglect their own basic medical care (Dunn et al. 2009; Gross et al. 2000), perhaps because of time pressure or because of concerns about confidentiality (Roberts et al. 2005). The message medical students receive tends to frame excellent patient care as potentially competing with good self-care. For example, the Accreditation Council for Graduate Medical Education (2018) professionalism guidance promotes "responsiveness to patient needs that supersedes self-interest" (p. 18), suggesting that self-care should be secondary, an idea that has deep historical roots in medicine (Trockel 2019).

In spite of these strong messages, powerful counterexamples have gradually begun to undermine the problematic view of the infallible doctor and suggest that the humanity of psychiatrists and psychologists can also be viewed as a potential source of strength. In part, this mind shift occurred because of individual physicians who wrote about their own illnesses and how the experience as patients made them more compassionate. In a compelling lecture titled "Arrogance," Franz Ingelfinger described the poignant experience of working as a doctor who eventually contracted a disease in which he was an expert. He outlined the confusion his family felt without guidance from an authoritative physician in whom they could place their trust. In the following provocative state-

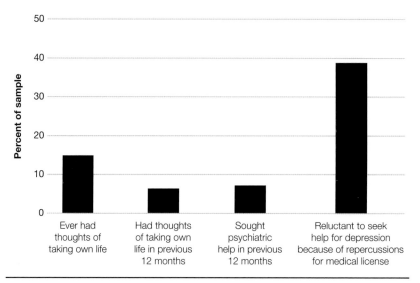

FIGURE 1–1. Suicidal ideation and reluctance to seek mental health care among American surgeons (*N*=7,905).

Source.   Data from Shanafelt et al. 2011.

ment, he imagined the benefits of restricting the practice of medicine to individuals who had been patients themselves.

> One might suggest, of course, that only those who have been hospitalized during their adolescent or adult years be admitted to medical school. Such a practice would not only increase the number of empathic doctors; it would also permit the whole elaborate system of medical-school admissions to be jettisoned. (Ingelfinger 1980, p. 1511)

After living through a significant medical illness, many physicians reflect on the ways in which they have treated patients in the past and wish they had done better. It is particularly striking that Ingelfinger noted in 1980 that the already growing pressures of efficient practice and computerized medical records were making personal relationships with patients, so necessary for effective care in his view, quite difficult. He concluded that the personal experiences of physicians inform their empathic practice. His writing had major influence on a generation of physicians struggling to reconcile their real-life experiences with the "good doctor" ideal.

System-level responsibility for sick doctors has been another galvanizing issue in the history of physician wellness. Many people believe that with all the self-sacrifice doctors commit for the sake of patient care, their institutions owe them, at a minimum, decent health coverage. Doctors who risk contracting serious illness in the line of duty provide an extreme example of this important issue. For instance, the case of Dr. Hacib Aoun, who in 1983 contracted HIV from a needlestick and was ostracized by his colleagues and dismissed from his hospital employment, sparked outrage about the treatment of sick physicians. In a *New York Times* article, Dr. Aoun described his poor treatment by colleagues and by his employer.

> "It is hard enough to live with the nightmare of AIDS, especially with a wife and a small child," Dr. Aoun said. "But to hear colleagues drop innuendos and issue slanderous comments about my private life and hear that the institution you committed yourself to will not help—that is too much." (Hiltsmarch 1990)

This case, and other similar experiences of stigma and inadequate care for physicians, prompted overdue improvements in institutional policy for injured doctors and, importantly, set the stage for more widespread physician health programs.

Inspired by stories like those of Franz Ingelfinger and Hacib Aoun as well as by the deeply personal experience of giving birth to her first child as a medical student, one of the authors (L.W.R.) began studying the health-related experiences of medical students and residents. This research revealed the tremendous stress associated with students or residents having any kind of health care need while in training. Students struggled with time demands, embarrassment, worries about access or costs of care, and awkwardness or vulnerability associated with the dual role of learner and patient, especially when seeking care in a training setting or from health care professionals who also served as teaching attendings. Students went to great lengths to obtain prescriptions from colleagues, mostly residents, "off the record." It became apparent, too, that the experience of being a patient while in training had a profound formative impact: there was a great deal more to learn about the importance of compassion, competence, and self-advocacy than any book could teach.

In interviewing other medical students across the country, it became clear that many medical schools did not require comprehensive health insurance, an issue that persists today, particularly for mental health and addiction treatment. Students at some institutions were extremely worried about their health, about becoming ill, about their ability to obtain health care, and about adverse repercussions for their careers should it be known that they needed, or sought, health services. These conversations prompted the first multi-institutional study of medical student health care in the United States (Roberts et al. 2000).

More than 1,000 medical students at nine medical schools participated in this initial survey project (52% response rate, with response rates varying from 20% to 87% by school) (Roberts et al. 2000, 2001). Nearly all students—93% women and 87% men—in the study had health care needs. Most students had deferred or avoided necessary health care because of confidentiality, cost, and time constraints. Students, especially women and clinical-level students, strongly preferred the option for care outside of the training institution. Students expressed concern that they would experience academic jeopardy, such as lower grades from supervisors or a negative letter from the dean's office for residency, particularly for stigmatizing health issues. These concerns were greater for women and for students identifying as members of an underrepresented minority. The narratives provided by respondents—about their own or their loved ones' illnesses—were extraordinarily moving.

Interestingly, in the 1990s, only a limited set of medical education journals and psychiatry journals were willing to publish papers on the topic of medical student and physician wellness. Viewing the topic as unimportant or, perhaps, as self-important, it was difficult to persuade most medical editors and peer reviewers of the salience and impact of the health and health practices of physicians and physicians-in-training.

Thus, another set of historical barriers to acknowledging the importance of physician wellness is the perception that doctors are a highly privileged group. In the context of the vast range of human suffering, it seemed self-centered to focus on the well-being of these "elites." Today, an emerging science of well-being—across fields of medicine, psychology, ethics, and organizational management—supports the idea that self-care is not selfish or overly indulgent but is critical for providing effective care (Baker 2003; Menon and Trockel 2019). In fact, the practitioner's state of mind has tremendous influence on medical decision-making. Therefore, cultivating the emotional literacy and mindfulness of psychiatrists and psychologists can help ensure that decisions are made after considering all relevant medical and psychological/contextual evidence. One example of this approach has been called *mindful practice* (Epstein 1999), which can help physicians act with compassion, solve difficult problems, and cope with emotional experiences that arise during practice.

In direct contrast to the problematic ideal of the superhuman doctor, a new image of health professionals is now emerging that is focused on improving wellness for both patients and physicians through common humanity and self-compassion (Horowitz 2019; Trockel 2019). Self-compassion means practicing mindfully and with kindness, not just with others, but with one's self as well (Neff and Germer 2013). The self-compassionate approach to physician wellness has taken many decades to emerge, but it offers great promise as an authentic way to move forward for both healthier patients and health care professionals.

From Avoiding Professional Burnout to Enhancing Professional Engagement

Burnout was first described in the 1970s to capture the experience of therapists who were feeling mentally and physically depleted and no longer functioning effectively (Schaufeli et al. 2009). As the study of this phenomenon has progressed, burnout has come to be known as a syndrome involving three components: emotional exhaustion, depersonalization, and perceived lack of personal accomplishment (Maslach and Jackson 1981) (Figure 1–2).

As the economies of many nations have shifted toward service sector jobs, burnout has emerged as a topic of great importance (Schaufeli et al. 2009). The risk of burnout increases when workload is excessive and workers have minimal control or inadequate rewards. Conflicting values, perceived inequities, and poor interpersonal communication in the workplace are also contributors (Leiter and Maslach 1999). Thousands of studies have now been published on the topic of burnout, and the World Health Organization has classified burnout in ICD-11 as a syndrome tied to "chronic workplace stress that has not been successfully managed" (World Health Organization 2018). Over the years, the study of professional burnout has contributed greatly to the understanding of factors that promote, and also detract from, professional fulfillment and life satisfaction.

There are also legitimate concerns that the emphasis on the burnout construct can overshadow several critical wellness issues. First, the construct of burnout may be used to describe a wide range of symptoms that warrant differential treatment. The seriousness of clinical depression or suicidality, for example, can be obscured by the use of such a broad term. Second, defining a negative outcome like burnout provides inadequate guidance about what optimal functioning should look like.

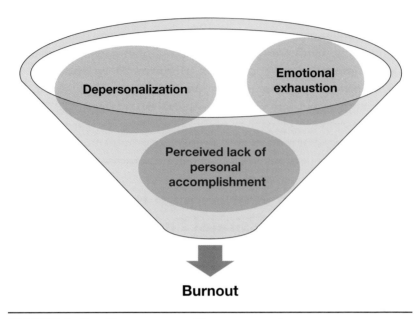

Burnout

FIGURE 1–2. Components of burnout syndrome.

The goal of avoiding burnout is now seen as just a small component of a more important positive objective: enhancing professional engagement. Defined in contrast to the burnout syndrome, *engagement* is evidenced by high energy, strong involvement, and increased sense of personal accomplishment (MacKinnon and Murray 2018). The positive psychology movement (Seligman et al. 2005) has further informed this transition from an emphasis on deficits and problems in the workplace toward exploration of opportunities for personal growth through meaningful work. Finally, the emphasis on clinician burnout can be criticized for placing implicit blame on the individual clinician, when, often, system-level drivers are major contributors to the prevalence of burnout. Improving clinician engagement and wellness (with associated decreases in burnout) will require a mind-set shift across many aspects of practice, ideally starting with early training experiences (Eckleberry-Hunt et al. 2009).

The Professional Fulfillment Index (PFI), proposed by one of the authors (L.W.R.) along with colleagues, was created to assess dimensions of well-being among health professionals in a brief but more positive and balanced manner than other instruments that focus primarily on negative feelings toward work (Trockel et al. 2018). The PFI seeks to evaluate variables that are relevant to physicians, measure change in response to workplace interventions, and uncover positive (fulfillment) and negative (burnout) aspects of health professionals' work. The PFI underwent testing and was found to correlate with existing measures of burnout, although it includes additional domains, such as experience with making mistakes and evolving feelings and attitudes over time. Initial empirical work with the PFI suggests that it may provide a valid and reliable new methodology to advance the field of physician well-being. Findings that derive from the use of the PFI may also help to determine whether efforts to strengthen individual well-being and to introduce systemic interventions make a constructive difference.

Costs of Clinician Burnout

One major reason that physician well-being matters is the relationship between psychiatrists' and psychologists' well-being and the quality of patient care. Evidence suggests that physician burnout is associated with more medical errors (Shanafelt et al. 2010; West et al. 2009). Studies of psychotherapists have also indicated that burnout is associated with lower quality of care (Lee et al. 2011; McCarthy and Frieze 1999). The depersonalization psychiatrists and psychologists may feel when experiencing burnout also diminishes capacities of empathy and conscientiousness, which are critical when caring for the mentally ill. Mismanagement of personal boundary issues can also compromise quality of patient care. For instance, a clinician who lacks close personal connections outside the workplace may be more vulnerable to engaging in inappropriate relationships with patients or colleagues.

Studies show that doctors are also more likely to recommend preventive health care strategies that they themselves actually use (Frank et al. 2013). Psychiatrists' and psychologists' practice of healthy behaviors may actually be one of the strongest predictors of whether they emphasize prevention with patients (Frank et al. 2000; Shahar et al. 2009), with data coming from diverse areas ranging from exercise to smoking cessation (Abramson et al. 2000; Howe and Monin 2017; Pipe et al. 2009). What this literature suggests is that the patients of doctors who practice poor self-care likely receive less guidance regarding health-promoting behaviors. In contrast, efforts to improve clinician health could have important downstream effects on patients' health.

Burnout and compromised well-being can also have significant business costs for organizations (as discussed in detail in Chapter 3, "Burnout and Clinician Mental Health," and Chapter 7, "Legal and Ethical Issues in the Context of Impairment and Recovery"). Across fields, when a psychiatrist or psychologist leaves the profession, the cost of replacing that individual in the workforce is significant. When psychiatrists and psychologists work with reduced efficiency, or call in sick frequently, the organizations they work for suffer. Burnout in mental health care can be especially problematic because of the relational nature of treatment (Lim et al. 2010).

Finally, the well-being of mental health care professionals can be seen as an ethical issue. First, self-care can be considered an ethical imperative related to competence (Wise et al. 2012). Psychiatrists and psychologists have an obligation to practice within the boundaries of competence, including seeking medical and mental health care for themselves when needed. In addition, mental health care professionals have a human right to strive for health and wellness, the same objective they pursue so passionately for their patients. As the medical field has increasingly embraced the importance of preventive health care strategies for patients, there is greater appreciation of the important role that prevention plays in promoting physician health as well. When psychiatrists and psychologists know about the suffering of their colleagues and trainees, they have an obligation to help. Taking steps to improve their wellness, whether small or large, is the right thing to do for the sake of patients, for the sake of colleagues, and for the sake of psychiatrists, psychologists, and future generations.

Individual and System-Level Interventions

In this book, we review a wide range of strategies for enhancing clinician well-being. These strategies include both system supports that can be put in place and practical approaches that individual psychiatrists and psychologists can employ in support of their own wellness. Because of the growing recognition that burnout is a symptom of organizational problems, rather than individual physician weakness (MacKinnon and Murray 2018), many types of system-level interventions have been proposed. For instance, workload and schedule adjustments, mentorship programs, and decision-making processes that allow for input from staff at all levels of the organization may help reduce burnout (Panagioti et al. 2017). In addition, a wide variety of innovative methods and programs have been proposed and tested to enhance system health and clinician engagement. These include changes in the way psychiatrists and psychologists document care, increased use of technology in treatment, regular opportunities for professionals to discuss wellness issues with peers, and leadership training programs. System-level interventions are discussed in detail in Chapter 6 ("Systems and Supports for Clinician Wellness").

For individual health care professionals, a wealth of practices can enhance well-being. In the final chapters of the book, we review down-to-earth advice for professionals seeking to enhance their own well-being. For instance, many physicians find that deliberately scheduling healthy activities helps them stay accountable for their own self-care. Burnout may make psychiatrists and psychologists more vulnerable to depression. Likewise, depression may make a person more vulnerable to burnout. Research has suggested that healthy activities, such as regular exercise, can help protect against these negative outcomes (Toker and Biron 2012). Work on meaningful projects also helps, including making a clear list of personal and professional priorities and feeling comfortable enough to say no to opportunities that do not advance worthy and personal goals. Routine medical care and mental health treatment as needed are critical for healthy functioning. Vacation and time for social connections also feed a full life. Exposure to nature helps many people recharge and combat mental drain experienced by overwork or stress (Berto 2014). Self-compassion is also critical so that real challenges can be acknowledged and addressed without harmful self-sacrifice.

Although mentorship and close connections with colleagues are critical for all professionals, the more isolated the psychiatrist or psychologist is during work, the more important strong mentorship relationships likely will be. Individuals in private practice must be uniquely responsible for their own self-care and burnout prevention (Lee et al. 2011) and must often take the initiative to self-evaluate and seek peer consultation and supervision as needed to perform patient care with competence. Mentoring is known to reduce the risk of burnout in academic faculty members (Van Emmerik 2004). In psychology, approximately two-thirds of Ph.D. students report having a mentor; the figure is lower for Psy.D. students (Clark et al. 2000). The low rates are particularly concerning given that mentor relationships established in graduate school often form the basis for mentoring relationships in early-career professionals, either because the mentor continues to support the individual after graduation or because the mentor is instrumental in connecting the individual with another important mentor relationship. Institutional recognition of faculty who excel at providing such support should be seriously considered as a system-level intervention to help incentivize staff to perform this critical role (Johnson et al. 2000).

Special Issues in Mental Health Care

Exposure to both acute psychiatric illness and chronic relational problems can place particular strain on the emotional well-being of mental health care professionals. The relationship between clinicians and their patients is by nature emotionally demanding (Lim et al. 2010). Psychiatrists and psychologists in this domain are exposed to a wide range of potentially difficult content, which puts them at risk for emotional depletion and secondary traumatization (Baker 2003; Lee et al. 2011).

A national survey of 285 therapists supported the idea that providing mental health care has significant influence on the mental state of health care professionals themselves (Pope and Tabachnick 1993). For instance, a large majority of therapists reported experiencing anger toward a patient at some point. More than half of the health care professionals reported at least one time when their own sleep, eating, or cognitive function was affected by their worry about a patient. Adding to the complexity of studying burnout in mental health care professionals is the fact that overinvolvement increases emotional exhaustion and depersonalization—key drivers of burnout. That same overinvolvement can also increase the psychiatrist's sense of personal accomplishment, which can mitigate burnout (Lee et al. 2011). Figure 1–3 depicts some of the key factors that draw physicians to the field of medicine and keep them motivated to practice (Ratanawongsa et al. 2006).

Mental health care professionals similarly often enter the field because of a deep sense of empathy and a strong wish to help others. The perfectionism necessary to succeed through many years of training may actually work against health care professionals once they enter practice. That is, the unmet needs of patients may be hard to ignore if a psychiatrist or psychologist is used to taking responsibility when a need arises. The conscientiousness necessary to dedicate one's life to service of others also makes these psychiatrists and psychologists uniquely vulnerable to overextending themselves. It may be hard to maintain appropriate boundaries with patients if their need seems great. If adequate resources are not available, health care professionals may feel under pressure to sacrifice their own sleep, family time, or other important tasks in order to provide care that will not be accessed otherwise (Lim et al. 2010). The qualities of perfectionism, conscientiousness, and empathy can also place practicing psychiatrists and psychologists at particular risk for becoming overextended or burned out, as illustrated in the following vignette.

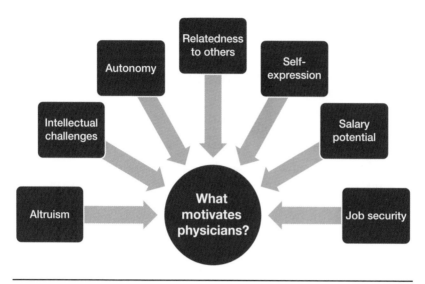

FIGURE 1–3.   What motivates physicians?

Source.   Adapted from Ratanawongsa et al. 2006.

Vignette

Ever since he was a child, Darnell Young was a good student and always prided himself in being helpful and responsible. As a medical student, these personal qualities helped him earn good grades and the respect of his fellow students and his teachers. But medical school was challenging, and he had to work hard to keep up with his classmates. He often stayed up all night writing, researching, and editing papers to make sure they were perfect. Many times, in his clinic rotations, he found that by working extra hours he could more easily complete the work. It felt good that his supervisors always praised him for being so conscientious.

Later, as a psychiatry resident, Dr. Young became known in his class for taking extra time, not just to take care of his patients but also to help any of his fellow residents if they were struggling. His willingness to go above and beyond and his empathy for his colleagues earned him the chief resident position in his final year, a role which made him very proud.

After finishing residency, Dr. Young started his first job as a psychiatrist in a community clinic. He soon had a full caseload and a number of important administrative duties. He wanted to provide outstanding care and to be viewed as a compassionate leader in the organization, but the work was more than one person could handle. Even though he was working overtime to try to handle all of the tasks, he soon found himself stretched too thin. The strategies he had used in medical school, such as staying up late to finish work, seemed insufficient to succeed in this new role. In addition, he had more trouble getting out of bed in the morning than he ever had. On some days, he felt so exhausted that he did not feel the same empathy for his patients that he usually felt. It seemed his work was not appreciated or making much of a difference anyway. He started to call in sick more frequently and even started thinking that he might have chosen the wrong career path.

Special Issues for Students and Trainees

A large body of evidence suggests that trainees and professionals in the earliest stages of their careers may be particularly vulnerable to burnout (Baker 2003). Young age is one of the factors most consistently associated with burnout (Lim et al. 2010), with multiple previous studies showing that older professionals are less likely to report emotional exhaustion than are younger professionals (Rosenberg and Pace 2006). As mental health professionals accumulate substantial work experience, they appear to be at lower risk for burnout (Lim et al. 2010).

It is concerning that medical students show higher rates of psychological distress than do age-matched peers, especially since they are a subgroup of individuals with many strengths and lower rates of burnout and depression before medical school (Baker and Sen 2016; Brazeau et al. 2014; Dyrbye et al. 2006). Students may also be less likely to seek care for medical or mental health problems because of fear of stigma or adverse academic or career consequences. For this reason, students need both easy access to confidential treatment and a culture that legitimizes self-care. Aspects of medical training that exacerbate symptoms of burnout and risk of psychiatric illness warrant change, even if major curricular and institutional modifications are needed to accomplish this (Slavin et al. 2014).

The process of becoming a doctor is a process of identity formation (Baker and Sen 2016). The training to become a medical professional or mental health care clinician brings serious risks. First, there are overt risk factors, such as long hours, heavy workload, sleep deprivation, financial strain, and mistreatment by authority figures. A hidden curriculum (Hafferty and Franks 1994) values an unrealistic ideal of perfectionism and self-sacrifice. Trainees are often taught that their suffering is a normal part of the process and that admitting to struggling is an unwelcome sign of weakness in a highly competitive environment. Table 1–2 summarizes the findings from a six-school study of depression and suicidal ideation in 2,193 physicians-in-training (Goebert et al. 2009). The data reveal a concerning trend that females experienced more frequent

TABLE 1–2. Depression and suicidal ideation in physicians-in-training

	Percent reporting either probable major depression or minor/moderate depression (*N*=1,883)	Percent reporting recent suicidal ideation (*N*=1,800)
All students	21%	6%
Gender[a]		
Male	16%	5%
Female	22%	6%
Ethnicity[b]		
Caucasian	22%	5%
Alaska Native, Native American, Pacific Islander	23%	16%
Black/African American	32%	13%
Hispanic	22%	8%
Asian	23%	6%

[a]For depression, *N*=1,723; for suicidal ideation, *N*=1,786. Not all respondents reported gender.
[b]For depression, *N*=1,089; for suicidal ideation, *N*=1,668. Not all respondents reported ethnicity.
Source. Adapted from Goebert et al. 2009.

depression symptoms, and ethnic minority students were at higher risk for suicidal ideation.

Evidence that students from underrepresented racial, ethnic, gender, and sexual minority groups are at substantial additional risk of depression (Hunt et al. 2015; Lapinski and Sexton 2014; Przedworski et al. 2015) is even more troubling. In their recent study of students enrolled in 49 different medical schools, Dyrbye and colleagues (2019) found that nonwhite students had significantly higher rates of depression. Although mentorship can be a critical ingredient for increasing both academic success and belonging, the persistent underrepresentation of faculty in academic medicine who identify as members of racial, ethnic, gender, and sexual minority groups means that students have minimal access to role models who may share critical aspects of their personal identities. Wellness programming should therefore include deliberate hiring of diverse staff and engagement of cultural consultants (Seritan et al. 2015). Physical health disparities are already closely linked to class and race. If wellness programming is primarily designed by and for majority culture individuals, there is a good chance it will fail to adequately address the unique needs of underrepresented minorities (Kirkland 2014).

Gender Differences and Caregiving Roles

The relationship between burnout and gender appears to be complex. Although many previous studies have documented equivalent levels of burnout across men and women (Lim et al. 2010; Thornton 1992), other studies have indicated that women may be at risk of emotional exhaustion, particularly when practicing within an agency (Rupert and Morgan 2005). Other recent surveys have documented that women physicians report burnout at significantly higher rates than men do (Shanafelt et al. 2012, 2016). On the other hand, a large meta-analysis of burnout in therapists indicated that male professionals were more likely to experience the specific category of burnout symptoms termed *depersonalization* (Lim et al. 2010), suggesting that the symptoms of burnout may manifest differently in men and women. Awareness of these potential differences can help supervisors and mentors to better monitor psychiatrists' and psychologists' well-being and intervene early.

Data from the American Time Use Survey suggest that women spend more time on average both completing household chores and taking care of other family members (U.S. Bureau of Labor Statistics 2015). Because women working full-time continue to bear substantial household maintenance and caregiving responsibilities in many families, the challenges of work-life balance can have particular potency for women. The role of parenting can also have substantial influence on wellness for both men and women, with differential effects depending on the extent of the individual's caregiving role and support system. Meeting the demands of raising healthy children while maintaining personal wellness and professional productivity can place a major burden on working parents, especially those who have lower income or are single parents (Kirkland 2014). To be effective, wellness interventions need to take into account both gender differences and differential caregiving roles. Psychiatrists and psychologists need programs and solutions tailored or individualized to meet their diverse needs. As illustrated in the following vignette, institutional wellness programming can be ineffective if a one-size-fits-all approach is taken.

Vignette

During her second year of psychiatry residency, Kara Price noticed she was feeling overwhelmed, unmotivated, and burned out. She spoke with the training director about her concerns. The director seemed familiar with the types of problems Dr. Price was reporting and gave her a packet of suggested resources. When Dr. Price arrived home, she realized she would not be able to take advantage of most of the programs. She had gained enough weight over the past few years that she was uncomfortable doing most of the physical exercise programs available through the university's wellness program. Also, as a single mother, she would not be able to attend any extra meetings or events without childcare. It seemed that when the programs had been designed, they had been tailored to an able-bodied, childless resident. Dr. Price started to feel even more hopeless and alone because the resources designed to help instead made her see how different she was from other residents.

Potential Problems With Wellness Programming

Wellness campaigns can be criticized for placing too much emphasis on a predetermined set of solutions and dismissing individual diversity. In fact, there are a wide range of viable solutions for enhancing the well-being of individual health care professionals. No particular set of solutions will be right for every professional. Although system supports are essential, engagement with wellness initiatives must be voluntary, selection of which activities to pursue must be individualized, and diverse perspectives on the desired outcomes must be respected. When making an effort to inspire groups of professionals to participate in activities to enhance wellness, great care must be taken to make sure campaigns do not become a new way to discriminate against people who have diverse life choices or development trajectories.

Aspects of both medical training and practice place psychiatrists and psychologists in particularly vulnerable positions. The nature of the work can feel isolating, and demanding schedules can limit the health care professional's ability to be in connection with loved ones. At times when the young person's developing identity is fragile, feedback systems can be designed to exploit this vulnerability to exact hard work and substantial personal sacrifice. Finally, the financial commitment required to complete training can add to the feeling that trainees are being exploited inappropriately. These factors contribute to the criticism that the field of medicine can feel like a cult at times. Although a growing emphasis on psychiatrist and psychologist well-being is an attempt to mitigate many of these problems, there is a risk that it can be one more form of unachievable perfectionism, placing too much of the blame on the individual health care professional already struggling to survive the pressures of a challenging job.

Kirkland (2014) makes a compelling case that institutions and leaders must be careful not to use wellness programming in a way that becomes discriminatory. In her article, Kirkland argues that wellness programming risks reproducing hierarchy and condoning discrimination based on personal health characteristics (Kirkland 2014). Wellness programs may reward those who are already healthy and risk having little impact on those who have few resources or are coping with substantial health problems. The fallacy that health is primarily under individual control can also lead to assumptions that individuals who are not healthy, for whatever reason, deserve their lower status. For individuals with disabilities, there is even greater risk that narrowly defined wellness programming will further exclude them. Although civil rights laws protect employees from discrimination based on personal characteristics, and employers ordinarily cannot legally discriminate on the basis of employee health status, employers are allowed to offer health coverage at a reduced cost contingent on employee achievement of specified health goals. Careful consideration of the ways in which wellness programming can exacerbate existing disparities and legal protections for a diverse workforce is strongly needed.

Another concern is that doctors who promote themselves as wellness experts may actually alienate patients who might be intimidated to discuss their shortcomings with someone perceived to be thriving under similar circumstances. In primary care, for instance, an overweight patient may be reluctant to visit a physician who appears to be thin or whose online profile boasts about regular exercise. Emerging evidence suggests that when physicians express an inclusive philosophy related to self-care that acknowledges individual differences and a nonjudgmental attitude, patients may feel more comfortable (Howe and Monin 2017). Although less is known about the extent to which this pattern is applicable to mental health care, it is reasonable to consider whether visible wellness activities of psychiatrists and psychologists may alienate patients who have psychiatric illness or significant relational problems. Certainly, inclusive messaging remains important in the mental health context.

Recognizing these pitfalls, the aim of this book is to take an authentic look at the important challenges related to professional wellness for psychiatrists' and psychologists' mental health care and to offer ideas for a self-compassionate approach to enhancing their well-being. Institutionally administered wellness programs may be harmful if they inadvertently isolate psychiatrists and psychologists who are already feeling vulnerable. A mindful approach dedicated to inclusivity and open listening is critical.

Positive Practices

1. Deliberately talk about self-care with colleagues and trainees. Demystify the process of integrating meaningful professional work and a fulfilling personal life. Share what you know and what has worked for you so far.
2. When you talk to patients about wellness activities, make an effort to use inclusive and nonjudgmental language.
3. Measure clinician engagement in your organization. Before developing an organizational strategy for improving clinician engagement, it is helpful to have data to understand the extent and nature of any existing problem with clinician burnout. It is therefore a recommended practice for organizations to gather data regarding clinician well-being on a regular basis to inform interventions and to benchmark progress. Find out if the organization where you work measures psychiatrists' and psychologists' engagement or symptoms of burnout on a regular basis. If not, what actions could you take to encourage accurate measurement of wellness in your organization?

Conclusion

The growing scientific interest in wellness is a reason for optimism about the health of psychiatrists, psychologists, and their colleagues. The study of systems under strain, as well as systems that appear to be functioning well, will help inform next steps for intervention. Continued development of innovative tools for measuring outcomes that really matter will also be essential. In spite of major methodological challenges, substantial progress is already being made in the study of physician wellness and the application of these lessons for a wide variety of mental health care professionals.

Questions to Discuss With Colleagues and Mentors

————————o————————

- What role does one's personal health and health care have in clinical training and practice?
- What do you think about the societal view of psychiatrists and psychologists as "superheroes"? Where does this idea come from, and what purpose does it serve? What other ways can we approach this issue in the health professions?
- What are the contributors to professional burnout? Who is most at risk, and why?
- What steps can we take to support good health and to address burnout before it starts?
- What are the special issues that mental health care professionals experience with self-care?

————————o————————

Recommended Resources

Brady KJS, Trockel MT, Khan CT, et al: What do we mean by physician wellness? A systematic review of its definition and measurement. Acad Psychiatry 42(1):94–108, 2018

Kirkland, A: Critical perspectives on wellness. J Health Polit Policy Law 39(5):971–988, 2014, 25037834

Lee J, Lim N, Yang E, Lee SM: Antecedents and consequences of three dimensions of burnout in psychotherapists: a meta-analysis. Prof Psychol Res Pr 42(3):252–258, 2011

MacKinnon M, Murray S: Reframing physician burnout as an organizational problem: a novel pragmatic approach to physician burnout. Acad Psychiatry 42(1):123–128, 2018

Roberts LW, Trockel MT (eds): The Art and Science of Physician Well-being: A Handbook for Physicians and Trainees. Cham, Switzerland, Springer, 2019

Thomas L, Ripp J, West C: Charter on physician wellbeing. JAMA 319(15):1541–1542, 2018

References

Abramson S, Stein J, Schaufele M, et al: Personal exercise habits and counseling practices of primary care physicians: a national survey. Clin J Sport Med 10(1):40–48, 2000 10695849

Accreditation Council for Graduate Medical Education: Common Program Requirements (Residency), 2018. Available at: https://www.acgme.org/What-We-Do/Accreditation/Common-Program-Requirements. Accessed December 24, 2018.

Baker EK: Caring for Ourselves: A Therapist's Guide to Personal and Professional Wellbeing. Washington, DC, American Psychological Association, 2003

Baker K, Sen S: Healing medicine's future: prioritizing physician trainee mental health. AMA J Ethics 18(6):604–613, 2016, 27322994

Berto R: The role of nature in coping with psycho-physiological stress: a literature review on restorativeness. Behav Sci (Basel) 4(4):394–409, 2014 25431444

Brady KJS, Trockel MT, Khan CT, et al: What do we mean by physician wellness? A systematic review of its definition and measurement. Acad Psychiatry 42(1):94–108, 2018 28913621

Brazeau CMLR, Shanafelt T, Durning SJ, et al: Distress among matriculating medical students relative to the general population. Acad Med 89(11):1520–1525, 2014 25250752

Clark RA, Harden SL, Johnson WB: Mentor relationships in clinical psychology doctoral training: results of a national survey. Teach Psychol 27(4):262–268, 2000

Dunn LB, Green Hammond KA, Roberts LW: Delaying care, avoiding stigma: residents' attitudes toward obtaining personal health care. Acad Med 84(2):242–250, 2009 19174679

Dyrbye LN, Thomas MR, Shanafelt TD: Systematic review of depression, anxiety, and other indicators of psychological distress among U.S. and Canadian medical students. Acad Med 81(4):354–373, 2006 16565188

Dyrbye LN, Wittlin NM, Hardeman RR, et al: A prognostic index to identify the risk of developing depression symptoms among U.S. medical students derived from a national, four-year longitudinal study. Acad Med 94(2):217–226, 2019 30188367

Eckleberry-Hunt J, Van Dyke A, Lick D, Tucciarone J: Changing the conversation from burnout to wellness: physician well-being in residency training programs. J Grad Med Educ 1(2):225–230, 2009 21975983

Epstein RM: Mindful practice. JAMA 282(9):833–839, 1999 10478689

Frank E, Rothenberg R, Lewis C, Belodoff BF: Correlates of physicians' prevention-related practices: findings from the Women Physicians' Health Study. Arch Fam Med 9(4):359–367, 2000 10776365

Frank E, Segura C, Shen H, Oberg E: Predictors of Canadian physicians' prevention counseling practices. Can J Public Health 101(5):390–395, 2010 21214054

Frank E, Dresner Y, Shani M, Vinker S: The association between physicians' and patients' preventive health practices. CMAJ 185(8):649–653, 2013 23569163

Goebert D, Thompson D, Takeshita J, et al: Depressive symptoms in medical students and residents: a multischool study. Acad Med 84(2):236–241, 2009 19174678

Gross CP, Mead LA, Ford DE, Klag MJ: Physician, heal thyself? Regular source
of care and use of preventive health services among physicians. Arch Intern
Med 160(21):3209–3214, 2000 11088080

Hafferty FW, Franks R: The hidden curriculum, ethics teaching, and the structure of medical education. Acad Med 69(11):861–871, 1994 7945681

Hiltsmarch PJ: Hospitals awaken to staff AIDS risk. New York Times, March 10,
1990. Available at: www.nytimes.com/1990/03/10/us/hospitals-awaken-
to-staff-aids-risk.html. Accessed August 23, 2019.

Horowitz R: Compassion cultivation, in The Art and Science of Physician Well-
being: A Handbook for Physicians and Trainees. Edited by Roberts LW,
Trockel MT. Cham, Switzerland, Springer, 2019, pp 33–56

Howe LC, Monin B: Healthier than thou? "Practicing what you preach" back-
fires by increasing anticipated devaluation. J Pers Soc Psychol 112(5):718–
735, 2017 28240939

Hunt JB, Eisenberg D, Lu L, Gathright M: Racial/ethnic disparities in mental
health care utilization among U.S. college students: applying the institution of medicine definition of health care disparities. Acad Psychiatry
39(5):520–526, 2015 25026942

Ingelfinger FJ: Arrogance. N Engl J Med 303(26):1507–1511, 1980 7432420

Johnson WB, Koch C, Fallow GO, Huwe JM: Prevalence of mentoring in clinical
versus experimental doctoral programs. Psychotherapy 37(4):325–334,
2000

Kirkland A: Critical perspectives on wellness. J Health Polit Policy Law
39(5):971–988, 2014 25037834

Lapinski J, Sexton P: Still in the closet: the invisible minority in medical education. BMC Med Educ 14(1):171, 2014 25128252

Lee J, Lim N, Yang E, Lee SM: Antecedents and consequences of three dimensions of burnout in psychotherapists: a meta-analysis. Prof Psychol Res Pr
42(3):252–258, 2011

Leiter MP, Maslach C: Six areas of worklife: a model of the organizational context of burnout. J Health Hum Serv Adm 21(4):472–489, 1999 10621016

Lim N, Kim EK, Kim H, et al: Individual and work-related factors influencing
burnout of mental health professionals: a meta-analysis. J Employ Couns
47(2):86–96, 2010

MacKinnon M, Murray S: Reframing physician burnout as an organizational
problem: a novel pragmatic approach to physician burnout. Acad Psychiatry 42(1):123–128, 2018 28247366

Maslach C, Jackson SE: The measurement of experienced burnout. J Organ Behav 2(2):99–113, 1981

McCarthy WC, Frieze IH: Negative aspects of therapy: client perceptions of therapists' social influence, burnout, and quality of care. J Social Issues
55(1):33–50, 1999

Menon NK, Trockel MT: Creating a culture of wellness, in The Art and Science
of Physician Wellbeing: A Handbook for Physicians and Trainees. Edited by
Roberts LW, Trockel MT. Cham, Switzerland, Springer, 2019, pp. 19–32

Neff KD, Germer CK: A pilot study and randomized controlled trial of the mindful self-compassion program. J Clin Psychol 69(1):28–44, 2013 23070875

Panagioti M, Panagopoulou E, Bower P, et al: Controlled interventions to reduce burnout in physicians: a systematic review and meta-analysis. JAMA Intern Med 177(2):195–205, 2017 27918798

Pipe A, Sorensen M, Reid R: Physician smoking status, attitudes toward smoking, and cessation advice to patients: an international survey. Patient Educ Couns 74(1):118–123, 2009 18774670

Pope KS, Tabachnick BG: Therapists' anger, hate, fear, and sexual feelings: national survey of therapist responses, client characteristics, critical events, formal complaints, and training. Prof Psychol Res Pr 24(2):142–152, 1993

Przedworski JM, Dovidio JF, Hardeman RR, et al: A comparison of the mental health and well-being of sexual minority and heterosexual first-year medical students: a report from the Medical Student CHANGE study. Acad Med 90(5):652–659, 2015 25674912

Ratanawongsa N, Howell EE, Wright SM: What motivates physicians throughout their careers in medicine? Compr Ther 32(4):210–217, 2006 17918306

Roberts LW, Warner TD, Carter D, et al: Caring for medical students as patients: access to services and care-seeking practices of 1,027 students at nine medical schools: Collaborative Research Group on Medical Student Healthcare. Acad Med 75(3):272–277, 2000 10724317

Roberts LW, Warner TD, Lyketsos C, et al: Perceptions of academic vulnerability associated with personal illness: a study of 1,027 students at nine medical schools: Collaborative Research Group on Medical Student Health. Compr Psychiatry 42(1):1–15, 2001 11154710

Roberts LW, Warner TD, Rogers M, et al: Medical student illness and impairment: a vignette-based survey study involving 955 students at 9 medical schools: Collaborative Research Group on Medical Student Health Care. Compr Psychiatry 46(3):229–237, 2005 16021594

Rosenberg T, Pace M: Burnout among mental health professionals: special considerations for the marriage and family therapist. J Marital Fam Ther 32(1):87–99, 2006 16468683

Rupert PA, Morgan DJ: Work setting and burnout among professional psychologists. Prof Psychol Res Pr 36(5):544–550, 2005

Schaufeli WB, Leiter MP, Maslach C: Burnout: 35 years of research and practice. Career Development International 14(3):204–220, 2009

Seligman MEP, Steen TA, Park N, Peterson C: Positive psychology progress: empirical validation of interventions. Am Psychol 60(5):410–421, 2005 16045394

Seritan AL, Rai G, Servis M, Pomeroy C: The office of student wellness: innovating to improve student mental health. Acad Psychiatry 39(1):80–84, 2015 24840666

Shahar DR, Henkin Y, Rozen GS, et al: A controlled intervention study of changing health-providers' attitudes toward personal lifestyle habits and health-promotion skills. Nutrition 25(5):532–539, 2009 19230614

Shanafelt TD, Balch CM, Bechamps G, et al: Burnout and medical errors among American surgeons. Ann Surg 251(6):995–1000, 2010 19934755

Shanafelt TD, Balch CM, Dyrbye L, et al: Special report: suicidal ideation among American surgeons. Arch Surg 146(1):54–62, 2011 21242446

Shanafelt TD, Oreskovich MR, Dyrbye LN, et al: Avoiding burnout: the personal health habits and wellness practices of US surgeons. Ann Surg 255(4):625–633, 2012 22388107

Shanafelt TD, Dyrbye LN, Sinsky C, et al: Relationship between clerical burden and characteristics of the electronic environment with physician burnout and professional satisfaction. Mayo Clin Proc 91(7):836–848, 2016 27313121

Slavin SJ, Schindler DL, Chibnall JT: Medical student mental health 3.0: improving student wellness through curricular changes. Acad Med 89(4):573–577, 2014 24556765

Thornton PI: The relation of coping, appraisal, and burnout in mental health workers. J Psychol 126(3):261–271, 1992 1527773

Toker S, Biron M: Job burnout and depression: unraveling their temporal relationship and considering the role of physical activity. J Appl Psychol 97(3):699–710, 2012 22229693

Trockel MT: Calling, compassionate self, and cultural norms in medicine, in The Art and Science of Physician Wellbeing: A Handbook for Physicians and Trainees. Edited by Roberts LW, Trockel MT. Cham, Switzerland, Springer, 2019, pp 3–17

Trockel M, Bohman B, Lesure E, et al: A brief instrument to assess both burnout and professional fulfillment in physicians: reliability and validity, including correlation with self-reported medical errors, in a sample of resident and practicing physicians. Acad Psychiatry 42(1):11–24, 2018 29196982

U.S. Bureau of Labor Statistics: American Time Use Survey, 2015. Available at: www.bls.gov/tus/charts/household.htm. Accessed August 23, 2019.

Van Emmerik H: For better and for worse: adverse working conditions and the beneficial effects of mentoring. Career Development International 9(4):358–373, 2004

West CP, Tan AD, Habermann TM, et al: Association of resident fatigue and distress with perceived medical errors. JAMA 302(12):1294–1300, 2009 19773564

Wise EH, Hersh MA, Gibson CM: Ethics, self-care and well-being for psychologists: reenvisioning the stress-distress continuum. Prof Psychol Res Pr 43(5):487–494, 2012

World Health Organization: QD85 Burn-out. ICD-11 for Mortality and Morbidity Statistics, 2018. Available at https://icd.who.int/browse11/lm/en#/http://id.who.int/icd/entity/129180281. Accessed July 16, 2019.

꩜

CHAPTER 2

Professional and Personal Developmental Milestones

W*ellness* refers to being in a good-quality state of health or being, typically subsequent to purposeful, consistent self-care behaviors. Professional wellness as a developmental construct emphasizes inherent fluidity of wellness and the potential for growth. Indeed, wellness is impacted by life experiences and may require consistent investment in self-care and access to reliable and thriving social support networks. Wellness can be expected to fluctuate over the course of an individual's life. For example, overcoming adversity, such as divorce or illness, profoundly affects an individual's concurrent emotional vulnerability, tolerance for professional responsibility, and ability to cope with future challenges. In addition, iterative professional development and subsequent advancement often yield new resources, such as personal resilience, a wider or more deeply connected professional network, authority in workplace decision-making, and greater financial stability.

Prevention of burnout is increasingly considered a core aspect of professional competence and ethical practice (Rupert et al. 2015; Wise et al. 2012) across the professional life span. Competent psychiatrists and psychologists are expected to cope effectively with personal challenges in such a way that they do not adversely affect their clinical work. For licensed psychologists, for example, the ethical code clearly specifies that psychologists "undertake ongoing efforts to develop and maintain their competence" and that when psychologists "become aware of personal problems that may interfere with their performing work-related duties adequately, they take appropriate measures" (American Psychological Association 2017). Similarly, policies are emerging to support physician health, and self-care has been considered by some organizations (e.g., the Royal College of Physicians and Surgeons of Canada and the United Kingdom's General Medical Council) to be a core competency for physicians (Seritan 2013).

The developmental perspective also acknowledges contextual variables strongly influencing wellness, including demographic factors, cultural practices, and gender-based expectations. For instance, although large numbers of studies show that both women and men report difficulty balancing the demands of family life and work, evidence shows that mothers may report slightly more family interference with work than do fathers (Shockley et al. 2017). Women may also face challenges to professional advancement.

In this chapter, we focus on the benefits of viewing professional wellness from a developmental lens and chronicle unique challenges faced by health care professionals at different stages of professional and personal development. Professional stages will be discussed first, followed by personal development related to major life events—marriage, divorce, child-rearing, and caring for aging parents. The professional trajectory of many psychiatrists and psychologists in academic settings, for example, goes through a natural evolution from training and early-career roles where the emphasis is on *demonstrating* promise to the later stages of professional life when the focus is on *fulfilling* promise. One example of a career progression in academic medicine is depicted in Figure 2–1.

Outside the academic setting, similar progression often occurs as experienced professionals take on leadership roles or have growing influence over programs in their organizations. In this chapter, we chronicle potential stressors as well as wellness growth opportunities relevant at different stages of professional development. Common experiences drawn from both faculty in academic medicine and psychiatrists and psychologists in other types of settings are highlighted.

Graduate Education: Medical School and Graduate School

Future psychiatrists begin their specialized training with medical school, typically receiving general medical education before specialized training in mental health issues. In contrast, in other fields such as psychology and social work, specialized training as a mental health care professional may begin at the start of the graduate school experience. In both cases, the experience of being a student brings unique challenges for cultivating

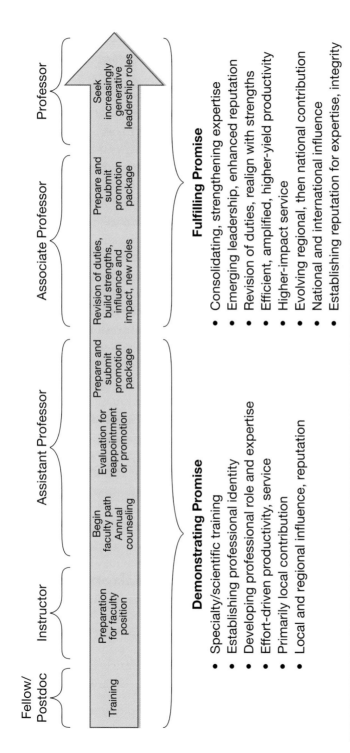

FIGURE 2–1. Example of career progression in academic medicine.

Source. Copyright 2005 by Laura Weiss Roberts. Reprinted with permission.

and maintaining wellness as well as many opportunities for professional growth (Table 2–1).

Stressors

Professional training in medicine and other mental health fields can be highly stressful because of academic pressures, financial burden, time pressure, and the need to apply classroom learning to in vivo clinical scenarios (Dyrbye et al. 2006; Matheson et al. 2016). Geographic separation from loved ones and heavy workload can further strain the trainee's vital social support network (Irving et al. 2009). Research suggests that many students may actually experience declining mental health over the course of their medical school enrollment. For instance, approximately 28% of medical students exhibit symptoms of depression (Puthran et al. 2016). Students also exhibit anxiety, suicidal thoughts, and substance abuse (Dyrbye et al. 2005). Similar challenges have been reported in graduate training programs for other mental health disciplines.

Access to effective treatment for trainees may be hampered by concerns about stigma, confidentiality, or negative educational or professional repercussions (Roberts et al. 2011). Medical students may even be encouraged to "tough it out" rather than seek care for their struggles (Baker and Sen 2016). Particularly concerning is the evidence from the annually administered Graduation Questionnaire on medical student health care issues from the Association of American Medical Colleges, which has indicated significant variability in wellness policies across U.S. medical schools and has highlighted troubling cultures of mistreatment in some cases (Baker and Sen 2016; Dyrbye et al. 2006).

Researchers have also hypothesized that students who choose to pursue medical or mental health training could have higher preexisting risk of depression or anxiety, making them potentially even more vulnerable to stress (Irving et al. 2009). The challenge of starting a career can also be particularly stressful for individuals who may be the first in their family to pursue higher education. The high cost of graduate education can exacerbate feelings of duress for this already vulnerable group of young people, as illustrated in the following vignette.

Vignette

Josepha Ruiz and Matt Stone are graduating medical students, getting married in 8 months, and both seeking residency spots in psychiatry. They were advised that being in the same residency program might not be ideal for their individual growth and learning. For this reason, they

TABLE 2–1. Common experiences and positive practices for medical and graduate students

Common experiences	Positive practices
• Extensive academic and clinical workload • High volume of new material • Family and friends do not understand • Remote social support network • Sense of urgency to "do something to help" • First-time vicarious traumatization • Sleep deprivation • Social isolation	**Talking to mentors:** Have career talks about what comes after graduate training in order to heighten enthusiasm and highlight pivotal transitions. **Self-care:** Explore options outside the university for self-care activities: • See a therapist • Join a hiking club • Take a yoga class **Familiarizing yourself with resources:** Any time a faculty member acknowledges that access to physical and mental health care is a necessary part of student life, the culture of support for student well-being is reinforced. • If supervising graduate or medical students, know about university- and community-based resources. • Routinely include resource information in student orientation materials so that this can also be subsequently emphasized at later points during training. • Post resource information on a student services website to make it widely accessible to students in need and easy to access in a confidential manner.

are looking at larger urban settings with more than one medical school and a number of psychiatry residency programs, hoping that these choices will optimize the chances of working in the same city, but not the same program, after medical school. On Match Day, they learn that they have both been assigned positions in a large metropolitan area—an area that is far from their families, is expensive, and has poor public transportation. As they approach the move to the new city, they determine that housing and transportation costs are roughly twice what they anticipated. They also discover that one of Matt's school loans must be paid off starting in residency, rather than after his training is completed. They both feel overwhelmed and filled with doubt. At graduation, Josepha confides to her mother, "This was supposed to be one of the happiest days of my life, and I just feel terrified."

Wellness Growth Opportunity

Graduate school can be a unique opportunity for early intervention and prevention of many later mental health challenges. Medical students and trainees are in the developmental process of beginning to cultivate their professional identities (Baker and Sen 2016). Personal and professional habits developed during this phase are likely to have an outsized effect on the individual's future professional development (Moutier 2013). In addition, data suggest that more than half of practicing psychiatrists still practice in the same state where they completed graduate medical education (Association of American Medical Colleges 2016), suggesting how important community connections established during graduate school can be over the professional life span.

Medical schools are now mandated by the Liaison Committee on Medical Education to educate students on topics related to well-being and stress management and to offer activities to enhance physical and mental health for students. Wellness programming embedded directly in the curriculum has also been suggested as a proactive strategy to enhance health during graduate medical training (Drolet and Rodgers 2010; West et al. 2014). Additionally, some physicians and educators have argued that medical school requirements should be redesigned so that they do less harm (Moir et al. 2018; Slavin et al. 2014). Solutions such as pass/fail grading systems have been proposed to reduce unhelpful competition and encourage students to support each other's learning and progress.

Many training programs are recognizing the need to expand community partnerships to support graduate student mental health. Although this can require administrators to negotiate with student health systems and insurance programs to allow care off campus, concerns about confidentiality and academic repercussions for seeking care mean that off-site resources are often the most comfortable option for students who need treatment. Even prevention activities can be arranged to be led by professionals outside of the core faculty. For instance, students might be more willing to participate in a mindfulness training offered by a community-based psychiatrist rather than one of their faculty members.

Advanced Training: Residency, Internship, Fellowship, and Postdoc

Advanced training for doctoral-level mental health care professionals takes the form of residency and fellowship for psychiatrists or internship and postdoctoral fellowships for psychologists. These years often involve intense clinical care experiences, with exposure to new types of cases and conditions. Advanced trainees often have opportunities to explore potential new specialty areas and may begin to focus on an area of particular professional interest. Although still supervised, advanced trainees become increasingly responsible for clinical decision-making; documentation; and, in some cases, training or supervision of students. This transitional period from trainee to professional presents a new type of strain. For instance, evidence suggests that mental health challenges first encountered in medical school can be exacerbated in residency (Baker and Sen 2016). For this reason, innovative programs have been introduced to enhance wellness during this period (Table 2–2).

Stressors

Substantial clinical workloads, long hours, extensive documentation requirements, and night or weekend calls can exacerbate stress during advanced training. Evidence suggests that as many as 77% of residents experience symptoms of burnout (Chaukos et al. 2018). The problem is also significant for advanced trainees in psychology, although the numbers are not quite as high.

Despite their advanced training, individuals remain "trainees" by designation and, therefore, are under direct supervision of doctoral-level mental health professionals. Although trainees may choose aspects of their training, many activities are still required, and the lack of choice or control over daily work experience can be a source of stress. Perceived lack of control is one of the most significant contributors to feelings of burnout and professional dissatisfaction (Maslach et al. 2001). In addition, residents and interns report a feeling of being alone, likely because

TABLE 2–2.   Common experiences and positive practices for advanced trainees

Common experiences	Positive practices
• Extensive clinical workload • Need to make in vivo clinical decisions with post hoc supervision • Pressures to decide about next job after training completion	**Control over schedule:** To the extent possible, allow residents to provide input into their own rotation and call schedules. • Within a resident class, it is likely that personal preferences and family circumstances will mean that a schedule that is burdensome for some trainees could actually work well for others. • Development of a system that, while remaining fair, also accommodates some personal preference can have positive effects on a trainee's sense of control and well-being. **Consultation groups:** A number of graduate psychology programs and residency programs have successfully arranged consultation or process groups for students. • These groups can be a helpful forum for students to seek and provide peer support and learn strategies for coping with the diverse physical, cognitive, and emotional demands of training and mental health care. • To preserve confidentiality, groups can be led by a community-based psychologist or psychiatrist who does not participate in other aspects of the educational program or academic evaluations.

they are sometimes expected to address challenging clinical situations on their own and to consult with supervisors afterward (Jibson 2013).

The experience of supervising medical students or graduate students can also be challenging for advanced trainees. Residents, interns, or fellows may be responsible for introducing students to many aspects of clinical care on their rotations. When residents feel under pressure or mistreated by supervisors, the experience can contribute to a toxic work environment for the medical students they supervise. Interns and postdoctoral fellows may also feel caught between their supervising psychologist and the graduate students or other trainees they are mentoring or supervising.

The issue of extensive work hours has been a long-standing consideration in the advanced training of medical residents. In 2003 and 2011, the Accreditation Council of Graduate Medical Education released policies designed to reduce resident sleep deprivation and fatigue to protect both patient safety and the health of advanced trainees (Baker and Sen 2016; Moutier 2013). These changes to duty hour requirements are some of the most widespread efforts to support resident wellness and highlight the relationship between the health of advanced trainees and the quality of the patient care they provide. Additional efforts beyond addressing work hours are clearly needed, and development of innovative programming to improve resilience for advanced trainees has therefore been the topic of a number of recent studies (Baker and Sen 2016). Several of these pilot programs appear to be well accepted by residents (Chaukos et al. 2018). Less has been published about supporting advanced trainees in psychology, but similar programs may also be helpful.

Financial concerns are another major issue for advanced trainees who may have substantial debt from medical or graduate school and who are still in a period of training when earnings are low, as illustrated in the following vignette.

Vignette

Regina Hart is a 33-year-old general psychiatry resident who chose to go to medical school after several years as an elementary school teacher. Recognizing the tremendous shortage of physician experts in the community where she has lived and worked throughout her life, she originally planned to subspecialize as a child and adolescent psychiatrist because she felt that it would be the best way to help children in distress. Her longtime partner is a teacher in an underserved urban community. Dr. Hart and her partner would like to start a family and purchase a condominium, but they both are struggling with education debt and cannot qualify for a standard mortgage. Dr. Hart has become convinced that she cannot pursue additional training. She reasons that she must enter practice as a general psychiatrist, feeling that she ultimately must choose between having a child with her partner or becoming a child psychiatrist.

Wellness Growth Opportunity

Residency, internship, or postdoctoral fellowship periods can be important times for self-evaluation related to self-care. Particularly for students who struggled to establish healthy habits in graduate school, advanced training is a critical time for the trainee to work out how to be professionally responsible and still manage to have adequate sleep, nutrition, exercise, and time with loved ones. Peer support can be a critical resource during this period. Whether in a formal consultation group or in an informal network of peers in the same cohort, having fellow trainees provide emotional support and share what they have learned can be invaluable.

The increasing specialization as training progresses offers opportunity to engage in personally meaningful work. As trainees explore areas of specialization, learning how to be a strong advocate for their own professional interests can be critical to their success. If a trainee has strong interest in a particular type of work, it is appropriate to ask potential mentors about opportunities to get more involved. A trainee can also ask about potential opportunities to attend conferences, give guest lectures, or assist in writing papers. This type of networking can help when it comes time to find a first job and can help establish colleague relationships that may be valuable throughout one's career.

Early Career

Once formal training is complete and an individual enters the professional world as an early-career professional, the career trajectory and experience may vary considerably depending on the chosen work environment. Some professionals will enter a role in which they continue to work alongside many colleagues who are also mental health professionals. Other early-career professionals may take positions in primary care settings, schools, or community agencies where they work with health care workers from other disciplines and may be the only mental health specialist. Feelings of isolation can certainly be exacerbated when the work environment does not include other mental health professionals; however, all early-career professionals will likely benefit from cultivating a rich network of colleagues and mentors.

Stressors

Evidence suggests that younger clinicians are at higher risk of burnout compared with individuals who have more experience (Shanafelt et al. 2012). Targeted strategies may be warranted for the early professional period (Panagioti et al. 2017). The particularly high risk of burnout reported for early-career faculty has several potential sources. On completion of formal training, the process of searching for a first job may cause strain. Whereas some individuals may have an opportunity to work close to family and friends, others may decide to pursue a job opportunity that takes them far from the places and people they know. The reality of having to pay back significant debt from schooling may start to set in, and the stark difference in financial stability compared with peers who have already been in the workforce for many years now can be a significant source of worry. The following vignette provides an example of a mental health professional pondering her financial future in comparison to fellow colleagues and how her concerns potentially could lead to burnout.

Vignette

Andi Trager is a 45-year-old psychologist who accepted a position at a Veterans Affairs (VA) hospital immediately after completing her postdoctoral fellowship. Dr. Trager comes from a military family and feels that her work is meaningful and an expression of her own patriotism. The first to become a doctor in her family, she has supported herself throughout college, graduate school, and fellowship. She is proud to have essentially no debt, but she does not have savings and has not been able to save toward retirement. Her father retired at a relatively young age because of chronic health issues, and lately she has been helping to pay her father's health care bills. Dr. Trager compares her financial situation with that of her peers who are working in other settings that are far more lucrative. She wonders whether she will "ever get ahead" if she remains at her job with the VA.

Identity development of the early-career professional can be a significant challenge, and the various perceived images of the "good doctor" can be overwhelming and confusing (Baker and Sen 2016). Some early-career faculty members may have difficulty establishing productive and sustained mentorship relationships (Becker and Yager 2013). The realities of the work may also be different from what the individual had imagined during training. Early-career professionals may experience doubts about choosing the right specialty or work environment. Moreover, many new psychiatrists and psychologists feel like imposters (the *imposter syndrome*) as they move into an attending role or provide supervision of trainees for the first time. Others may experience external discrimination for being "too young." Early-career professionals may also find that the self-sacrifice strategies that worked for getting through training (Ratanawongsa et al. 2007) are not sustainable in the long term (Irving et al. 2009). Finally, similar to students and trainees, studies show that physicians in practice often avoid necessary health care because of fear of negative repercussions for their career, including threat of losing their license to practice, losing professional standing, or missing opportunities for advancement.

Wellness Growth Opportunity

Mentorship is critical, regardless of career stage, and the early-career period in particular is a time when professionals need strong mentorship (Table 2–3). A true *mentor* is someone who is senior, knowledgeable about areas of direct interest, and available and willing to be a sounding board and/or provide honest and trustworthy advice. The mentor should be able to meet on a regular basis to discuss the iterative critical decisions that help mold the career of the person being mentored. Often, mentors make introductions or provide opportunities that would not otherwise be immediately available without their direct influence.

In academic medicine, mentorship has been historically conceptualized as a core partnership in personal and professional development. With long hours and administrative, research, and other clinical demands placed on faculty of all career levels, establishing and sustaining a consistent mentor relationship can often prove challenging. A systematic review published in *JAMA* noted that less than 50% of medical students and, in some areas of clinical expertise, less than 20% of faculty members reported having a mentor (Sambunjak et al. 2006). Despite these modest figures, the sample endorsed mentorships' influence in multiple arenas, including career advancement, research productivity (i.e., publication and grant success), and personal development.

Just as mentorship can benefit early-career faculty by increasing career satisfaction and productivity (Palepu et al. 1998; Sambunjak et al. 2006), mentorship can also enhance a sense of professional community in the workplace for early-career professionals practicing outside academic medical settings. Psychiatrists and psychologists should consider seeking several mentors with distinct expertise. For instance, professionals find it helpful to have one or more technical mentors who can teach spe-

---

TABLE 2–3.   Benefits of mentorship

Mentors act in a wide variety of ways, often including but not limited to the following:

- Encouraging more contribution to the department
- Inviting the person being mentored to help with projects
- Writing letters of recommendation or reference for promotion or application for an award or other funding opportunity
- Being willing to introduce colleagues and opportunities that could prove fruitful in a project pipeline
- Discussing research and publication ideas
- Sharing information about their journey
- Advocating; being an ally
- Offering advice and a meaningful collegial relationship

---

cific skills or tasks. This type of relationship may be more time-limited and domain-specific. A developmental mentor may also be a wise choice. This individual is usually a more senior colleague who may not have expertise exactly aligned with the mentee's interest area but who is generally knowledgeable about how to build a successful career trajectory in the field of choice. A developmental mentor may also be personally committed to helping the mentee grow and progress (Borus 2013).

As the mentee's needs evolve over the course of his or her career, mentorship relationships also change. Having multiple professional mentoring relationships with diverse contributions (*mosaic mentoring*) may be best for supporting career growth (Becker and Yager 2013; Borus 2013). Seeking mentors with long-standing positive reputations and admirable interpersonal qualities may be helpful. For example, a good mentor might be someone who demonstrates collegial qualities in how he or she talks and works with others. Although productive mentoring relationships can take time to establish, developing a meaningful relationship with a supportive mentor can be beneficial throughout one's career.

Institutional support for finding appropriate mentorship varies across settings. In academic medical settings, for example, a mentor may be "assigned" at the outset of hiring. In other situations, programmatic infrastructures (e.g., research training grants that require mentorship) may be in place that match employees to a mentor with aligned research interests or areas of expertise. Other instances require that the mentor or mentee take the initiative to find a match. In this case, leveraging social networks within conferences, within a department, and within professional societies and clubs is a practical way to encounter potential mentors or mentees.

Peer mentoring can also be particularly helpful for early-career professionals. Emerging evidence suggests that peer mentoring can be a powerful way to support academic productivity and advancement for faculty (Becker and Yager 2013; Johnson et al. 2011). If working for a large organization, psychiatrists and psychologists should recruit colleagues internally. If working in a small organization, health care professionals can reach out to colleagues in other agencies or in private practice. Groups focused on both clinical consultation and professional development can be an important source of professional support. Regardless of the group composition, professionals find great satisfaction from helping others become established in their careers.

Many professional organizations or specialty societies have begun efforts to enhance involvement and supports for early-career members. When joining professional organizations, psychiatrists and psychologists should look for networks that may have pathways for early-career professionals to become involved. Special events at an organization's annual conference, such as mentoring programs and social gatherings, can be a good start. Some funding opportunities also give preference for early-career individuals. In some organizations, committee membership by early-career professionals is explicitly encouraged. For instance, the American Psychological Association and the American Psychiatric Association have made specific efforts to include early-career members on committees. Table 2–4 outlines both challenges and potential positive actions for early-career professionals.

Mid Career

The practice of mental health care is a type of work that can be continued for many decades, as is evident from available workforce data. For instance, the 2016 Physician Specialty Data Report suggested that more than 60% of active psychiatrists were age 55 or older (Association of American Medical Colleges 2016). A mid-career professional can contribute to well-being by amassing substantial experience and building a robust professional network. The mid-career period can be a time of both stability and change. There may be an increasing responsibility within a given job, or a mid-career professional may transition to a new organization or type of work. The effect of transitions on well-being can depend on whether the transition is perceived as a positive career move or a move made from necessity (e.g., to fill gaps in clinical or research op-

TABLE 2–4. Common experiences and positive practices for early-career professionals

Common experiences	Positive practices
• Learning systems in a new workplace • Practicing without supervision for the first time • Extensive clinical workload • Formally supervising residents or fellows • Unknown criteria for promotion • Paying off debt	**Networking:** The more contact you have with professionals doing similar community work, the more supported you will feel. • Seek out and meet other clinicians who endorse similar areas of specialty training; leverage these colleagues' expertise as questions about patients arise. • When relocating to a new geographic area or if a new job involves a patient population or type of care that is unfamiliar, develop a strong network of colleagues; this will feel like a lifeline. • Take the time to set up meetings with other mental health clinicians. • Ask for recommendations of colleagues who might have similar professional interests and systematically work to expand your network. • If feeling too busy, set a realistic goal for regular contact even if it is small (e.g., decide if one new lunch appointment per month or per quarter is manageable). **Peer mentorship:** Learn many of the skills necessary for a new job from peers who are also in the early stages of their career. • Do not be afraid to ask for help, and ask colleagues how they have learned to accomplish work-related tasks. • Offer similar mentorship in exchange. **Paying off educational debt:** Ask supervisor(s) and peers what their loan repayment plans are; start to sketch out how and when necessary payments can be made.

erations) (Jibson 2013). Changes in life circumstances over the course of a professional's career can mean changes in career goals, interests, and trajectory. Both job demands and personal responsibilities may be different during this period than they were during training or will be in the future (Table 2–5).

Stressors

Many mental health professionals have substantial caregiving responsibilities during the mid-career period, whether caring for their own children, aging parents, or both. These responsibilities have significant effects on both men and women, particularly those who have young children or are single parents, although women with substantial caregiving responsibilities may be under particular stress (Bergman et al. 2008; Seritan 2013). Burnout may have a particular effect on professionals in the mid-career stage. Some professionals choose to work part-time to accommodate family needs. Data on the physician workforce suggest that many more women than men work part-time or report intending to reduce from full-time to part-time work (Shanafelt et al. 2009).

Wellness Growth Opportunity

Mid career is a period when many professionals take on more leadership roles within their organizations. There may be times when there are many referrals, resulting in easily finding new patients. At other times, it is necessary to find new ways to spread the word about one's expertise, whether through face-to-face meetings with potential referral sources or through enhancing Web presence or other forms of advertising. In academic medicine, advancement may depend on establishing a strong clinical reputation locally, regionally, or nationally. The reputation is demonstrated through reliable high-quality clinical work, as well as such activities as public speaking, teaching, committee work, or publishing research.

Mid career is a great time to seek out and invest in administrative roles. New roles can offer fantastic opportunities to hone critical interpersonal skills, such as networking, collaboration, management, organization, and/or advocacy. Indeed, many faculty promotion tracks encourage and outright look for evidence of administrative initiative. A wide variety of administrative roles may exist within a department or in professional societies and association affiliations. Psychiatrists and psychologists can look for posted opportunities in newsletters, quarterly updates, or blogs and at annual meetings. Alternatively, health care professionals can seek

TABLE 2–5. Common experiences and positive practices for mid-career professionals

Common experiences	Positive practices

• Expanded responsibility at work
• Strong wish to do work that is meaningful
• Critical evaluation of own career choice
• Balancing research and clinical endeavors
• Taking on additional teaching responsibility
• Caregiving for children and/or aging parents
	Informing yourself: Make sure to explicitly ask about promotion requirements to understand what it will take to be successful in the organization.
	  • Keep track of completed activities to show advancement in leadership roles and your impact in the workplace.
	  • Be sure to document engagement in research, clinical, teaching, and publication activities, as well as any relevant volunteer and community service roles.
	Teaching: Teaching others can provide great personal and professional satisfaction. As a mid-career professional, you have substantial experience you can share with colleagues.
	  • Share your knowledge through either formal teaching or informal consultation.
	  • Volunteer to give a lecture for a class or professional organization, start a work group in your organization for professionals interested in learning about a specific topic, or develop online content that you can post on your website or share with interested colleagues.
	  • If you have difficulty figuring out topics to share with others, think broadly about the many aspects of your professional role.
	  • Share experience with a particular treatment technique or patient population.
	  • Consider sharing what you have learned about a wide range of other tasks (e.g., academic writing, political advocacy, budgeting, clinical supervision, any other topic about which you feel passionate).

opportunities to take an administrative lead on projects that have not yet been noticed as a department-wide need. Especially if the role is unpaid, thoughtful integration of administrative roles into one's workflow is imperative for long-term utility and survival.

A mid-career mental health professional may find that having one administrative role that is multipurpose may be helpful. For example, acting as a liaison to another department is an administrative role that can also serve as an opportunity for budding research collaboration between aligned faculty members from each department. Another sometimes unforeseen benefit of administrative roles is that they can boost professional and interpersonal skills as well as interdepartmental networks and collaborations. Such opportunities may diversify a professional's portfolio of skills while simultaneously helping to establish a niche and domain expertise.

Late Career

Development and milestones in the late period of a professional's career can vary greatly. Some older workers maintain substantial professional responsibilities. In fact, one of the benefits of mental health care as a professional specialty is that many psychiatrists and psychologists can continue practicing competently late into life. Indeed, psychiatry is recognized as the specialty with the third oldest demographic in the United States; in 2013, 46% of psychiatrists were older than age 65 (Brenner et al. 2017). Some professionals may partially reduce their workload to allow for personal, family, or community activities, whereas others may retire fully and pursue another type of work, volunteer activity, or leisure. Regardless, aging professionals face unique challenges (Table 2–6).

Stressors

Depending on workplace policies, there may be a formal process of assessment or peer evaluation for older employees to document cognitive fitness to continue practice. Even when professionals are not experiencing physical or mental decline relevant to their work performance, older adults may experience discrimination in the workplace. In the late-career period, health conditions may prevent continued practice or make reduction in work time or work responsibilities necessary. Decisions about retirement plans are often complicated by financial uncertainty. Some professionals are reluctant to retire because of worries that they may not have sufficient funds saved to adequately cover their living expenses and lifestyle.

TABLE 2–6.	Common experiences and positive practices for late-career professionals	

Common experiences	Positive practices
• Continuing to receive and provide mentorship • Advanced administrative or leadership roles • Establishing legacy • Preparing for retirement	**Mentorship:** By this career stage, you may already have substantial experience with mentoring. 　• Take time to consider which types of mentoring relationships have been most meaningful. 　• Consider whether your leadership or administrative expertise may allow you to mentor someone in a more senior role in addition to mentoring students or early-career faculty. **Legacy:** What should be done in this career phase to increase the chances that one of the programs in which you are involved is sustainable after retirement? 　• When reviewing professional roles and contributions, focus particularly on programs that have potential to be maintained long term. 　• Consider establishing a funding stream or training interested colleagues to run the program.

Wellness Growth Opportunity

Professional well-being is enhanced when clinicians spend a portion of their work time engaged in an activity with personal meaning. In a study of physicians of different ages, the data suggested that whereas physicians in the early-career and mid-career period spend equivalent amounts of time engaged in an activity of personal meaning, physicians in the later stages of their careers spend the most time engaged in work that is personally meaningful (Shanafelt et al. 2009). Many professionals also spend a portion of their late career providing substantial leadership to organizations or in their communities.

Serving as a mentor can be a powerful way to give back to the professional community and have a meaningful and lasting impact. The mentor may experience great personal or professional fulfillment from the chance to help a future leader develop and succeed in his or her chosen career path, and organizations can also incentivize and reward good mentorship. For instance, some institutions give awards for active mentors, and other institutions may formally track mentorship activities and use this information when making promotion decisions (Borus 2013).

When evaluating retirement options, professionals may consider a plan for partial retirement to be attractive as a transition from full-time work to full-time retirement. A period of partial retirement can be a way to focus primarily on work activities that have strong meaning for the individual and to simultaneously begin additional volunteer or leisure activities that will be prominent after full-time retirement. Making the transition gradually can help with adjustment to a new stage of life.

Personal Development

As psychiatrists and psychologists mature professionally, their personal lives develop in parallel. Each of these life stages are characterized by particular pressures and concerns.

Stressors

During medical or graduate school, and well into early-career stages, for example, mental health clinicians may be entering new relationships or exiting long-term romantic partnerships, having and rearing children, and becoming an integral part of a social community outside of the professional environment. Later years often involve considerations of physical and mental health care for an aging parent and/or losing a parent. Of course, no one is immune to an aging body, preparing for and facing retirement, and planning financially for well-being in the remaining years. Sometimes, as shown in the example below, life presents significant unexpected stressors, such as divorce or a chronic physical health condition within the immediate family.

Vignette

Paul Chan is a 43-year-old psychologist with a thriving private practice. He and his husband have two school-age children. His private practice schedule allows him a degree of flexibility, so he volunteers in his children's classrooms, which brings both him and the children joy and creates fond memories. His mother, Rina Chan, is single and lives on her own nearby. Ms. Chan enjoys spending time with her grandchildren and often enthusiastically helps Dr. Chan and his husband with childcare. Unexpectedly, Ms. Chan had a terrible fall and broke her hip. Suddenly, Dr. Chan was catapulted into the world of elder care, a completely new space for him. He felt as though he were enrolled in a crash course on skilled nursing options, interfacing with an entire care team who were managing various aspects of his mother's injury and recovery, reading the fine print about Medicare coverage, and, all the while, talking with his children about their grandmother's fall and her expected recovery. The accompanying financial burden was, although temporary, still significant. Dr. Chan realized that even though he himself was a health care professional, this specific realm was foreign and overwhelming. Dr. Chan rearranged much of his schedule to allow him the time to visit his mother during her surgery and hospitalization, drive her to and from physical therapy, and help with chores around her home. He reduced his volunteer hours at his children's school, and, for time's sake, reduced the frequency of cooking at home in exchange for serving prepared dinners.

Dr. Chan brought up his overwhelming stress within the context of his weekly consultation group, who had known and worked alongside him for more than a decade. One team member offered words of support and shared that his own father recently received a diagnosis of early-onset dementia and that he, too, struggled to learn rapidly about elder care, settings of care, and progressive diagnoses. The exchange of reciprocal and genuine empathy between Dr. Chan and his colleague was meaningful. It also provided an opportunity for him to reflect that he was not alone in caring for an elderly parent. He was grateful that his colleague had shared his own family struggles as well.

Wellness Growth Opportunity

A large portion of this book is dedicated to the discussion of the frank importance of self-care (e.g., social support, psychiatric care, physical activity, sleep). Caring for oneself through major life events is certainly no exception. Mental health clinicians are encouraged to seek out and talk with not only family and friends but also trusted colleagues, consultation groups, and mentors about navigating major life events in the context of attempting to propel one's career forward. Professionals working in a large organization can consider contacting their human resources department to learn about benefits, such as family medical leave. Starting conversations early, when possible, can facilitate the discovery or identification of resources to assist. Vulnerability in sharing about a major life event can lead to more opportunities to garner empathy and support from others, as well as the potential learning that can result when a close colleague describes managing a similar situation.

Grief

Loss is not an unusual experience for people in health professions. Loss may touch a clinician's life personally during the many years of training and practice. When the loss is unexpected or sudden, the experience of grief may be further complicated by the devastating impact of trauma. When a clinician-patient seeks psychological support after an acute loss, professionals should consider the emotional, social, cognitive, physical, and spiritual aspects of experiencing that loss (Pospos et al. 2018; Zisook et al. 2014). In speaking with the clinician-patient, psychiatrists and psychologists should ask the name of the person who has died and about the relationship with the deceased. Offering empathy and inquiring about how the clinician-patient is doing is important. The treating clinician should avoid making statements that could be experienced as unfeeling, isolating, or distancing, such as "I completely understand," "You will be fine in time," or "Time cures all." Psychiatrists and psychologists can sit quietly with the clinician-patient who is living with grief and moving through the pain of the experience of bereavement. Being present, kind, nonpathologizing, and nonjudgmental in the therapeutic interaction with a grieving individual is essential. Talk therapy may be valuable, and other experiences, such as exercise, massage, or animal therapy, also can play an important role in healing after a significant loss.

When grief has persisted for a long period and there is evidence of impairment or limitations in everyday function beyond the first few months, a potential diagnosis of complicated grief should be explored. Complicated grief is underrecognized, especially in older adults and in the aftermath of traumatic death (e.g., suicide, murder, sudden death, accident), and can have serious consequences for survivors. These consequences include loss of independence, diminished physical or mental health status, loss of identity, and the emergence of symptoms (e.g., suicidal ideation or impulsivity), particularly when the individual also has a co-occurring condition (e.g., mood or anxiety disorders or addiction). Each of these issues should be evaluated and appropriate treatment introduced. Waiting for complicated grief to resolve does not reflect a correct standard of psychiatric care.

Conclusion

Although personal well-being and professional productivity can seem at odds, engaging in meaningful work is a critical aspect of personal wellness. Competent practice and professional progress (i.e., career advancement, promotion, professional success) can also be a sign of wellness and effective work-life integration. When an individual can find personal professional interests that also benefit the organization or department where that professional is employed, meaningful work can be highly compatible with career advancement. Successful professionals seek growth opportunities that are aligned with both personal interests and initiatives of high value to their organization.

Similarly, self-care is critical for professional effectiveness. Acquiring the self-knowledge necessary to balance a competing set of personal priorities is a normal part of adult development. Although every stage of a professional's life may bring both unique stressors and growth opportunities, the earlier in the career that effective self-care is established, the more meaningful and lasting impact that professional can have. For this reason, addressing wellness challenges during training can have particularly potent long-term effects. When a young person makes progress, whether by figuring out how to work in regular exercise, how to prioritize both professional milestones and personal social connections, or how to treat the self with compassion even when work or life circumstances are challenging, the lifelong benefits can be substantial. Any intervention that makes graduate students and early-career professionals more skilled at caring for their own well-being can affect not only their current lives and current patients but also their future colleagues and trainees.

Questions to Discuss With Colleagues and Mentors

—————○—————

- What kind of advice did you find most helpful in your career so far?
- What strategies have you used to make sure your work is personally meaningful?
- What unique strengths do you think I can draw on in my career?
- What do you see as major areas where I need to grow professionally?
- Are there specific skills you think I should learn?
- Where can I learn more effective leadership skills?

—————○—————

Recommended Resources

Baker K, Sen S: Healing medicine's future: prioritizing physician trainee mental health. AMA J Ethics 18(6):604–613, 2016

Becker A, Yager J: How to approach mentorship as a mentee, in The Academic Medicine Handbook: A Guide to Achievement and Fulfillment for Academic Faculty. Edited by Roberts LW. New York, Springer, 2013, pp 157–162

Borus, JF: How to be a good mentor, in The Academic Medicine Handbook: A Guide to Achievement and Fulfillment for Academic Faculty. Edited by Roberts LW. New York, Springer, 2013, pp 163–169

Brenner AM, Balon R, Coverdale JH, et al: Psychiatry workforce and psychiatry recruitment: two intertwined challenges. Acad Psychiatry 41(2):202–206, 2017

Brown B: Daring Greatly: How the Courage to Be Vulnerable Transforms the Way We Live, Love, Parent, and Lead. New York, Avery, 2015

Dweck C: The power of believing that you can improve (video). November 2014. Available at: www.ted.com/talks/carol_dweck_the_power_of_believing_that_you_can_improve. Accessed July 17, 2019.

Dweck C: Mindset: The New Psychology of Success. New York, Ballantine, 2016

Jibson MD: How to strengthen your own and others' morale, in The Academic Medicine Handbook: A Guide to Achievement and Fulfillment for Academic Faculty. Edited by Roberts LW, New York, Springer, 2013, pp 343–354

Moir F, Yielder J, Sanson J, Chen Y: Depression in medical students: current insights. Adv Med Educ Pract 9:323–333, 2018

Moutier C: How to have a healthy life balance as an academic physician, in The Academic Medicine Handbook: A Guide to Achievement and Fulfillment for Academic Faculty. Edited by Roberts LW. New York, Springer, 2013, pp 429–435

Ofri D: What Doctors Feel: How Emotions Affect the Practice of Medicine. Boston, Beacon, MA, 2013

Roberts LW, Hilty DM (eds): Handbook of Career Development in Academic Psychiatry and Behavioral Sciences, 2nd edition. Arlington, VA, American Psychiatric Association Publishing, 2017

Seritan AL: How to recognize and avoid burnout, in The Academic Medicine Handbook: A Guide to Achievement and Fulfillment for

Academic Faculty. Edited by Roberts LW. New York, Springer, 2013, pp 447–453

Transue ER: On Call: A Doctor's Days and Nights in Residency. New York, St Martin's Griffin, 2004

References

American Psychological Association: Ethical principles of psychologists and code of conduct, 2017. Available at: www.apa.org/ethics/code/index. Accessed July 17, 2019.

Association of American Medical Colleges: Active physicians by age and specialty, 2015, from Physician Specialty Data Report, 2016. Available at: www.aamc.org/data/workforce/reports/458494/1-4-chart.html. Accessed August 12, 2019.

Baker K, Sen S: Healing medicine's future: prioritizing physician trainee mental health. AMA J Ethics 18(6):604–613, 2016 27322994

Becker A, Yager J: How to approach mentorship as a mentee, in The Academic Medicine Handbook: A Guide to Achievement and Fulfillment for Academic Faculty. Edited by Roberts LW. New York, Springer, 2013, pp 157–162

Bergman B, Ahmad F, Stewart DE: Work family balance, stress, and salivary cortisol in men and women academic physicians. Int J Behav Med 15(1):54–61, 2008 18444021

Borus JF: How to be a good mentor, in The Academic Medicine Handbook: A Guide to Achievement and Fulfillment for Academic Faculty. Edited by Roberts LW. New York, Springer, 2013, pp 163–169

Brenner AM, Balon R, Coverdale JH, et al: Psychiatry workforce and psychiatry recruitment: two intertwined challenges. Acad Psychiatry 41(2):202–206, 2017

Chaukos D, Chad-Friedman E, Mehta DH, et al: SMART-R: a prospective cohort study of a resilience curriculum for residents by residents. Acad Psychiatry 42(1):78–83, 2018 29098597

Drolet BC, Rodgers S: A comprehensive medical student wellness program—design and implementation at Vanderbilt School of Medicine. Acad Med 85(1):103–110, 2010 20042835

Dyrbye LN, Thomas MR, Shanafelt TD: Medical student distress: causes, consequences, and proposed solutions. Mayo Clin Proc 80(12):1613–1622, 2005 16342655

Dyrbye LN, Thomas MR, Shanafelt TD: Systematic review of depression, anxiety, and other indicators of psychological distress among U.S. and Canadian medical students. Acad Med 81(4):354–373, 2006 16565188

Irving JA, Dobkin PL, Park J: Cultivating mindfulness in health care professionals: a review of empirical studies of mindfulness-based stress reduction (MBSR). Complement Ther Clin Pract 15(2):61–66, 2009 19341981

Jibson MD: How to strengthen your own and others' morale, in The Academic Medicine Handbook: A Guide to Achievement and Fulfillment for Academic Faculty. Edited by Roberts LW. New York, Springer, 2013, pp 343–354

Johnson KS, Hastings SN, Purser JL, Whitson HE: The Junior Faculty Laboratory: an innovative model of peer mentoring. Acad Med 86(12):1577–1582, 2011 22030756

Maslach C, Schaufeli WB, Leiter MP: Job burnout. Annu Rev Psychol 52(52):397–422, 2001 11148311

Matheson KM, Barrett T, Landine J, et al: Experiences of psychological distress and sources of stress and support during medical training: a survey of medical students. Acad Psychiatry 40(1):63–68, 2016 26223316

Moir F, Yielder J, Sanson J, Chen Y: Depression in medical students: current insights. Adv Med Educ Pract 9:323–333, 2018 29765261

Moutier C: How to have a healthy life balance as an academic physician, in The Academic Medicine Handbook: A Guide to Achievement and Fulfillment for Academic Faculty. Edited by Roberts LW. New York, Springer, 2013, pp 429–435

Palepu A, Friedman RH, Barnett RC, et al: Junior faculty members' mentoring relationships and their professional development in U.S. medical schools. Acad Med 73(3):318–323, 1998 9526459

Panagioti M, Panagopoulou E, Bower P, et al: Controlled interventions to reduce burnout in physicians: a systematic review and meta-analysis. JAMA Intern Med 177(2):195–205, 2017 27918798

Pospos S, Young IT, Downs N, et al: Web-based tools and mobile applications to mitigate burnout, depression and suicidality among healthcare students and professionals: a systematic review. Academic Psychiatry 42(1):109–120, 2018 29256033

Puthran R, Zhang MWB, Tam WW, Ho RC: Prevalence of depression amongst medical students: a meta-analysis. Med Educ 50(4):456–468, 2016 26995484

Ratanawongsa N, Wright SM, Carrese JA: Well-being in residency: a time for temporary imbalance? Med Educ 41(3):273–280, 2007 17316212

Roberts LW, Warner TD, Smithpeter M, et al: Medical students as patients: implications of their dual role as explored in a vignette-based survey study of 1027 medical students at nine medical schools. Compr Psychiatry 52(4):405–412, 2011 21683176

Rupert PA, Miller AO, Dorociak KE: Preventing burnout: what does the research tell us? Prof Psychol Res Pr 46(3):168–174, 2015

Sambunjak D, Straus SE, Marusic A: Mentoring in academic medicine: a systematic review. JAMA 296(9):1103–1115, 2006 16954490

Seritan AL: How to recognize and avoid burnout, in The Academic Medicine Handbook: A Guide to Achievement and Fulfillment for Academic Faculty. Edited by Roberts LW. New York, Springer, 2013, pp. 447–453

Shanafelt TD, West CP, Sloan JA, et al: Career fit and burnout among academic faculty. Arch Intern Med 169(10):990–995, 2009 19468093

Shanafelt TD, Boone S, Tan L, et al: Burnout and satisfaction with work-life balance among US physicians relative to the general US population. Arch Intern Med 172(18):1377–1385, 2012 22911330

Shockley KM, Shen W, DeNunzio MM, et al: Disentangling the relationship between gender and work-family conflict: an integration of theoretical perspectives using meta-analytic methods. J Appl Psychol 102(12):1601–1635, 2017 28749157

Slavin SJ, Schindler DL, Chibnall JT: Medical student mental health 3.0: improving student wellness through curricular changes. Acad Med 89(4):573–577, 2014 24556765

West CP, Dyrbye LN, Rabatin JT, et al: Intervention to promote physician well-being, job satisfaction, and professionalism: a randomized clinical trial. JAMA Intern Med 174(4):527–533, 2014 24515493

Wise EH, Hersh MA, Gibson CM: Ethics, self-care and well-being for psychologists: reenvisioning the stress-distress continuum. Prof Psychol Res Pr 43(5):487–494, 2012

Zisook S, Iglewicz A, Avanzino J, et al: Bereavement: course, consequences, and care. Curr Psychiatry Rep 16(10):482, 2014 25135781

꙳ ꙳

CHAPTER 3

Burnout and Clinician Mental Health

The antithesis of well-being is *burnout*, a state of professional depletion characterized by exhaustion, cynicism, and a loss of meaning (Blackwelder et al. 2016). The term has an academic definition as well as idiosyncratic use cross-culturally, colloquially, and individually. If professional passion is the bright, steady internal flame of the inspired care worker, then burnout is the metaphorical smothering and eventual snuffing out of that flame over time as a result of chronic work stress. First coined in the early 1970s, burnout was originally conceptualized as comprising three components: emotional exhaustion, depersonalization, and a decreased sense of personal accomplishment (Maslach and Jackson 1981). These three components have been more broadly described as dimensions:

> The exhaustion dimension was also described as wearing out, loss of energy, depletion, debilitation, and fatigue. The cynicism dimension was originally called depersonalization (given the nature of human services occupations), but was also described as negative or inappropriate attitudes towards clients, irritability, loss of idealism, and withdrawal. The inefficacy dimension was originally called reduced personal accomplishment, and was also described as reduced productivity or capability, low morale, and an inability to cope. (Maslach and Leiter 2016, p. 103)

Specifically, burnout results when demands outstrip resources, leading to a gradual erosion of energy, idealism, and efficacy (Shanafelt et al. 2012). Since Maslach's early research, attention to the concept has grown exponentially in both the professional and public vernacular, with more than 6,000 publications on burnout published by the turn of the century (Schaufeli et al. 2009). Increasingly, the expression *burn(ed) out* has become, much like the term *stress*, a ubiquitous shorthand for the everyday experience of trying to keep up with one's fast-paced, modern life. The World Health Organization has classified burnout as a syndrome resulting from chronic workplace stress (World Health Organization 2018); including a more detailed definition of burnout in ICD-11 may result in increased awareness of and attention to the signs and symptoms of burnout, with doctors trained in the assessment and treatment of the condition.

Despite leading to serious and alarming consequences for health care professionals and the public, burnout is so widespread that it has become casual office vernacular, often used in a way that implies inevitability and the impossibility of solution. The implication is an accepted pervasiveness of the condition that belies its seriousness. In this chapter, we review the prevalence, risk factors, and potential outcomes of burnout as well as more significant mental health difficulties, including risk of suicide in mental health professionals.

Models of Burnout

Maslach and Jackson (1981) first identified the three-part model of burnout on the basis of their research with social service workers in California. Research supports this model and demonstrates that the three components of burnout operate sequentially, beginning with emotional exhaustion, leading to cynicism about the value of one's field or one's capacity to effect change, and finally culminating in disengagement and reduction in perceived personal accomplishment (Figure 3–1) (Schaufeli et al. 2009). Burnout is additionally defined in idiosyncratic ways, however, invoking only parts of the tripartite model. Cross-culturally, the term is sometimes used by researchers and theorists to indicate the exhaustion phase alone. At other times, the term refers only to an extreme version of the third phase. Burnout is differentiated colloquially from distress in that both involve impairment of professional functioning, but the former leads to long-term loss of the professional role, whereas the latter implies mild symptoms and only partial role impairment (Blackwelder et al. 2016).

Prevalence of Burnout

Medical and mental health professionals are at elevated risk for burnout. Burnout is higher for doctors at all levels of training than for any other profession, including other positions involving rigorous training leading to advanced professional degrees (Shanafelt et al. 2012). More than half of all practicing physicians report being burned out (Shanafelt

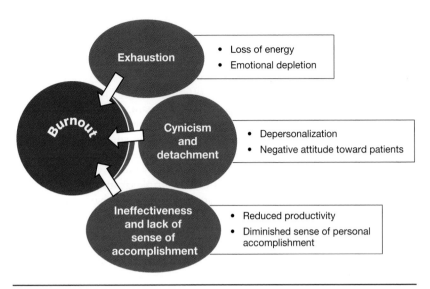

FIGURE 3–1. Dimensions of burnout.

et al. 2015), and burnout appears to begin during the training years. Prior to beginning schooling, medical students endorse lower rates of psychological distress than general population, age-matched control subjects. By completion of training, medical students have higher rates of distress than their peers (Brazeau et al. 2014). Comparably, more than 40% of nurses report occupational burnout (Vahey et al. 2004), and 60% of psychologists acknowledge significant depression at some point during their careers and working when they were too distressed to be effective (Barnett et al. 2007). Half of all psychotherapists across professional degrees (e.g., family therapists, social workers) endorse burnout (Simionato and Simpson 2018). Clearly, the issue is pervasive, and trends are worsening over time. Rates of both burnout and depression in medical professionals increased 0.5% annually from the 1980s to the present, despite targeted efforts by the Accreditation Council for Graduate Medical Education to reduce burnout (Shanafelt et al. 2015). The following example illustrates the case of a health professional who is on the verge of burnout.

Susceptibility to Burnout

Case Example 1

Alicia Carey is a recently relocated psychiatric nurse in her first year of work at a publicly funded hospital in her new home city. She is passionate about her clinical practice focused on supporting underprivileged families with high rates of trauma and historically limited access to care. She is inspired by the hospital's dedication to serving the local community and to enhancing health care for the low-income, substantially crime-exposed, and largely Latino community.

Ms. Carey is part of a small team offering bilingual mobile trauma treatment services for women. On joining the team, she throws herself into the effort, ecstatic to have a core group of like-minded colleagues. The team works long hours and most weekends to support a community of individuals who are often unable to take time off from work to seek services. Because the program is publicly funded, there is additional paperwork to complete, including multiple treatment planning documents, financial justification forms, and clinical progress demonstrations. Demand for the service is high, the wait lists are long, and the caseload is large.

The patients have limited resources themselves, and Ms. Carey finds herself frustrated by the few supports she can provide in the way of pragmatic needs, such as childcare, bus fare, low-income housing application support, and well-woman services. Her team lacks a social worker, and she often thinks fondly of the inspiring social workers at her former job. She vows to do what she can based on what she has observed and learned from social workers and spends time after hours conducting research on housing programs and job support services.

The supervisor is empathic but cautions Ms. Carey against doing extra work, warning that it is likely to burn her out. She knows her supervisor is right but reasons that if she does not continue, no one else will, and she cannot see patients in such need without trying to help. She finds it particularly challenging when families no longer qualify for publicly funded services and she is forced to discharge them from the program. Her patients tell her she is their only social support. She realizes there are limited alternatives she can offer outside her program. The programs she offers tend to have long wait times in the outpatient clinics and copays that outstrip resources.

As the caseload and the extent of patients' needs grow, Ms. Carey feels increasingly frustrated and hopeless. She begins to avoid her paperwork, and she has a sinking feeling in the pit of her stomach when she is referred a new patient because she knows she will not be able to help as much as she hopes. Then, rumors begin swirling around the hospital that the program may cease to exist entirely because of budget cuts. Employees are assured that they will not be laid off; however, the mobile unit programming is likely to be cut. Ms. Carey feels exhausted and overwhelmed. She does not want to leave her agency, but she wonders if a role reassignment will still allow her to serve the population of women to which she is committed.

Alicia Carey's position makes her susceptible to burnout. Although she finds her work deeply meaningful, the demand for services is high, the hours are long, and resources are insufficient. The administrative burden consumes a great deal of her energy, and suggestions by management to limit her after-hours contributions are at odds with her values—both of which are risk factors for burnout. Her deep investment in working with a highly traumatized population is a prime example of the intricate interplay between helpful and harmful elements of work. High levels of involvement with her patients' struggles can both provide meaning and lead to overinvolvement and contribute to greater burnout. The risk for the latter is higher because of the lack of sufficient resources to adequately address her patients' struggles.

The colleagues on Ms. Carey's small team offer social support and peer mentorship, providing a strong protective mechanism. However, the lack of administrative support from the larger organization and funding challenges confer risk. Although Ms. Carey and the organization share the same core value of helping the underserved community, they are moving further apart as the hospital confronts budget cuts and discontinues extra services, such as mobile crisis units. Being reassigned to another program would dramatically change Ms. Carey's role; reduce her sense of autonomy over her work; and, again, increase risk for burnout. Her feelings of frustration and hopelessness, along with avoiding administrative demands and feelings of dread in the pit of her stomach, are all symptoms of burnout's exhaustion phase.

The root causes for Ms. Carey's burnout risks are systemic, and an optimal solution could come at the level of institutional reform. The hospital's leadership may benefit from consultation to help consider alternatives to cutting values-consistent programming, such as a programmatic grant or donor funding; use of physician extenders, such as social workers and nurse practitioners; and a culture of support to reduce burnout systemically. Ms. Carey could benefit from greater mentorship from senior colleagues, who might help her think about how to advocate for the program she loves, how to shape her career, and how to follow her professional passions in this challenging scenario marked by high demand and limited resources.

Identifying and Measuring Burnout

Although multiple measures of burnout exist, the Maslach Burnout Inventory (MBI; Maslach and Jackson 1981) has held the dominant position as an instrument for assessing physician burnout and is used in greater than 90% of the existing studies on burnout (Schaufeli et al. 2009). The MBI is a validated 22-item self-report measure with three subcomponents that reflect the original definition of burnout (Shanafelt et al. 2012). The instrument is not freely available. The MBI has some overlap with measures of mood and anxiety conditions, which has introduced many challenges. The MBI is not immune from social desirability bias associated with self-report measures. Significant criticism has targeted the MBI's ambiguous and overly "generic" features and its evolving terminology. For instance, the original instrument referred to measuring *cynicism* as one dimension of burnout, and cynicism was then supplanted by the term *depersonalization*, which has an entirely different meaning in psychiatry and psychology literature.

Alternatives to the MBI are typically selected for feasibility of administration, to spare either financial cost or time (Maslach and Leiter 2016). A new instrument, the Copenhagen Burnout Inventory (CBI), has been developed and introduced to the public domain and has been integrated into the empirical study of burnout. The CBI is intended to measure much more precisely the dimensions of personal burnout, work-related burnout, and patient-related burnout. The CBI includes questions such as "How often do you feel tired?" and "How often do you think, 'I cannot take it anymore?'" to assess personal burnout. Additional questions to assess work-related burnout are "Do you feel worn out at the end of the working day?" "Does your work frustrate you?" "Are you exhausted in the morning at the thought of another day at work?" "Do you find it hard to work with clients?" and "Does it drain your energy to work with clients?" The CBI has been tested in a number of highly stressful settings, including prisons and hospitals in Europe (Kristensen et al. 2005). Although the CBI does appear to have greater attunement to the context of work, it may have some of the same problems as the MBI, including social desirability biases and a lack of clear, crisp separation from underlying mental health concerns.

Identifying the point at which burnout is reached is difficult and, to some degree, arbitrary. Unlike a pathogenic disease state, in which a condition is either present or absent, burnout, like other psychological variables, is continuous in nature. Because continuous variables make it difficult to answer practical questions, such as whom to treat or in which cases to pay out disability claims, many studies of burnout identify cut points to label employees with and without the condition and/or to divide them into severity groups (e.g., high, moderate, low burnout). Like other psychological variables of interest, burnout develops as a gradual process over time. Recognizing the continuous nature of burnout allows health care professionals to address a number of existing challenges to its prevention and amelioration, including the tendency to locate the concern in the individual, to stigmatize burnout as an illness or sign of vulnerability, and to assume that the natural state is the absence of burnout. Table 3–1 illustrates the Stanford Professional Fulfillment Index can be used to quantify burnout as well as professional fulfillment.

Costs of Burnout

Clinician Well-Being

Burnout is linked to a wide array of negative health outcomes for the individual, including increased rates of depression (Tennant 2001), suicide (Dyrbye et al. 2008), problematic alcohol use, somatic complaints (e.g., gastrointestinal issues, chronic pain, headaches, flu-like symptoms, insomnia) (Blackwelder et al. 2016), and relationship breakup (Shanafelt and Noseworthy 2017; Shanafelt et al. 2003). Preliminary work suggests that burnout may also be a precursor to depression. In one study, nearly all residents experiencing depression were also suffering from burnout, although not all residents suffering from burnout were also experiencing depression (Tennant 2001).

Patient Care

The cost to patients is vast when a medical professional is burned out (Shanafelt et al. 2012). Patients are affected at every level, from diagnosis to treatment to recovery, with poorer treatment experiences and worse outcomes when physicians, nurses, social workers, and therapists are burned out (Blackwelder et al. 2016; Schaufeli et al. 2009). Clinician burnout is associated with reduced adherence by patients to treatment plans, more medical errors, missed changes in patients' conditions (Bodenheimer and Sinsky 2014), and assessment of poorer care provision (Barnett et al. 2007). Burned-out clinicians exhibit lower empathy for patients (Vahey et al. 2004), and patients report lower satisfaction when treated by a burned-out professional (Bodenheimer and Sinsky 2014). Patients are also at risk for lengthy recoveries, greater mortality, and poorer prognoses (Trockel et al. 2018).

Organizational Losses

Employers are also hurt by clinician burnout. Motivation, retention, and performance are all negatively impacted by burnout (Wilson et al. 2017). Absenteeism, presenteeism (coming to work despite illness or burnout), turnover, and early retirement are higher (Kahill 1988; Shanafelt et al.

TABLE 3–1. Stanford Professional Fulfillment Index (PFI)

How true do you feel the following statements are about you at work during the past two weeks?	Not at all true Score=0	Somewhat true Score=1	Moderately true Score=2	Very True Score=3	Completely true Score=4
a. I feel happy at work	[]	[]	[]	[]	[]
b. I feel worthwhile at work	[]	[]	[]	[]	[]
c. My work is satisfying to me	[]	[]	[]	[]	[]
d. I feel in control when dealing with difficult problems at work	[]	[]	[]	[]	[]
e. My work is meaningful to me	[]	[]	[]	[]	[]
f. I'm contributing professionally (e.g., patient care, teaching, research, and leadership) in the ways I value most	[]	[]	[]	[]	[]

During the past two weeks, I have felt...	Not at all Score=0	Very little Score=1	Moderately Score=2	A lot Score=3	Extremely Score=4
a. A sense of dread when I think about work I have to do	[]	[]	[]	[]	[]
b. Physically exhausted at work	[]	[]	[]	[]	[]
c. Lacking in enthusiasm at work	[]	[]	[]	[]	[]
d. Emotionally exhausted at work	[]	[]	[]	[]	[]

TABLE 3–1. Stanford Professional Fulfillment Index (PFI) *(continued)*

During the past two weeks, my job has contributed to me feeling…	Not at all Score=0	Very little Score=1	Moderately Score=2	A lot Score=3	Extremely Score=4
a. Less empathetic with my patients	☐	☐	☐	☐	☐
b. Less empathetic with my colleagues	☐	☐	☐	☐	☐
c. Less sensitive to others' feelings/emotions	☐	☐	☐	☐	☐
d. Less interested in talking with my patients	☐	☐	☐	☐	☐
e. Less connected with my patients	☐	☐	☐	☐	☐
f. Less connected with my colleagues	☐	☐	☐	☐	☐

Note. Scoring for the PFI should be considered continuous—a higher score on burnout is negative, while a higher score on professional fulfillment is positive. However, suggested cut-points are also included below:

Professional fulfillment: add items 1–6 and divide by 6. Fulfillment > 3.0.

Burnout: add items 7–16 and divide by 10. Burnout > 1.33.

Source. Copyright 2016 Board of Trustees of the Leland Stanford Jr. University. All rights reserved. Nonprofit organizations are permitted to use this survey instrument without modification for research or program evaluation exclusively. An electronic version of the survey is available by contacting wellmdcenter@stanford.edu. Any other use of this survey is granted by express written permission of the Stanford WellMd Center by contacting wellmdcenter@stanford.edu.

2012), and performance is lower. Resources are overused, resulting in cost increases (Bodenheimer and Sinsky 2014). Physicians and therapists who are burned out are more likely to leave their positions, leading to clinician shortages. Staff shortages fuel a cycle of being underresourced and increasing burnout for remaining staff. Turnover costs are considerable, with estimates suggesting that replacing a single physician costs from $250,000 to $300,000 and represent more than 5% of a medical organization's costs (MacKinnon and Murray 2018). Additional organizational revenue is lost as a result of patient dissatisfaction, consequently harming the facility's reputation and brand.

Threats to Health Care Reform

As psychiatrists and psychologists attempt to resolve the nation's problems of insufficient medical insurance, rising health costs, and inadequate access to care, they are forced to confront the consequences of burnout. Dyrbye and Shanafelt (2011) highlight the very factors that increase risk for burnout, explaining that they are part and parcel of health care reform efforts. Demand outstripping resources is at the heart of burnout, and the goal of increasing access to care will only put greater demand on an already insufficient workforce. Higher costs of care and efforts to reduce margins are also predicted to place further pressure on psychiatrists and psychologists to do more with less. As oversight by insurance companies and other payers increases, so, too, do documentation and reporting requirements, which represent an additional administrative demand and are a common contributor to medical professional burnout. Efforts to solve access problems need to be considered carefully so as not to replace one challenge with another. For instance, use of nurses and physician extenders may reduce burnout for psychiatrists, but this may run the risk of transferring burnout to these other providers in the absence of systemic organizational change.

Antecedents and Causes

Individual Factors

Burnout has traditionally been viewed as a person-level variable (Maslach and Goldberg 1998), and, as such, the search for vulnerabilities and explanatory causes has been located in the individual employee. The belief that burnout reflects a personal failing is widespread in medicine, with a full 25% of residents erroneously believing that burnout was reportable to the medical board (Chaukos et al. 2017). There are, in fact, provider variables that correlate with burnout, including being younger and earlier in one's career (Simionato and Simpson 2018), having high levels of perfectionism and self-blame (Lee et al. 2011), and becoming deeply and emotionally invested in patients (Simionato and Simpson 2018). However, these variables are hardly personal failings. Emotional investment in patients is necessary for good care. Effective health professionals are empathic and emotionally invested in their work, and they are exposed daily to a painful side of life, hearing patients' stories and bearing witness to their struggles. As a result, overidentification and vicarious trauma are common in the helping professions (MacKinnon and Murray 2018). There is a complex relationship between being empathically invested and being overinvested. Particularly challenging for the health care clinician is the feeling of not being effective when patients fail to get better despite best efforts. "Constant caring without the compensation of success" (Lee et al. 2011) appears to more strongly incite burnout, as explained in the following in-depth example.

Case Example 2

Isabelle Kirkwood is a newly minted physician who is in the third month of her first year (i.e., internship) of her general psychiatry residency. During her third year of medical school, her father died from cancer, and she experienced a major depressive episode. She sought treatment and was able to complete medical school after a leave of absence, during which she engaged in personal psychotherapy and worked as a research assistant. She initially took an antidepressant that was effective for her major depression; she was able to taper and discontinue the antidepressant medication during her fourth year of medical school as she recovered.

The first 2 months of her internship consisted of working alongside a collegial group of psychiatry residents on an inpatient unit, and she felt supported and excited, despite the increased responsibilities of being an intern. Now she is rotating on an internal medicine service as part of a team that includes interns and residents from the internal medicine residency training program.

Because of Dr. Kirkwood's experience with her father's illness, caring for patients with serious medical illnesses is both profoundly moving as well as emotionally painful for her. After her first 3 weeks rotating on the internal medicine service, during which she is on overnight call every 5 nights, she begins to experience detachment and exhaustion. Although she is able to function adequately on the service, she feels emotionally depleted. On her days off, she stays in bed most of the time, feeling physically and mentally exhausted. Although she is aware that her symptoms are similar to feelings she experienced during her previous episode of depression, she also notices some differences. Specifically, she does not feel sad but does experience irritation at the many demands of her role in the hospital. Each patient feels like a burden, and she has difficulty empathizing with them and with their families. Her roommate, who is also a psychiatry intern, encourages her to consider talking to their program director about her symptoms.

Burnout shares symptom overlap with depression, as highlighted in this scenario. Although depression and burnout often share a subjective experience of exhaustion and withdrawal from previously meaningful activity, burnout is focused in the professional domain and is conceptualized as being in direct response to work demands that exceed resources. Burnout is reflected in Dr. Kirkwood's scenario, in which she feels depleted as opposed to sad and is resentful of the multiple competing demands of her internship role. A sudden lack of empathy toward patients could be a symptom of depression. For Dr. Kirkwood, however, the origins appear directly linked to her intensive call schedule and the personal nature of her work. The intersection of individual and systems contributions is also seen here. The experience of supporting her father through his medical illness is both a benefit and a risk because it adds an additional layer of meaning to Dr. Kirkwood's rotation in internal medicine and deepens the importance of the work. Her experience with her father's illness also sets up a risk for burnout to the extent that Dr. Kirkwood deeply identifies with her patients, intensifying the emotional workload. It is important to acknowledge the role of personal contributions (in this case, the historical loss of Dr. Kirkwood's father to cancer) without overlooking systemic factors, such as Dr. Kirkwood's intensive caseload, challenging patient population, and heavy call schedule. Because burnout can often be a precursor to depression, seeking support from her program director would be wise.

Although early-stage burnout is not the same as clinical depression, the conditions share many similar features. Table 3–2 outlines how symptoms of burnout can overlap with symptoms of major depression as well as key differences that set the conditions apart. If untreated, burnout can become severe and conveys significant risk for clinical depression and other psychiatric problems. In addition, individuals with a history of major depression, such as Dr. Kirkwood, may have heightened risk for burnout symptoms and may need additional supports to effectively cope with work-related stressors.

Organizational and Environmental Contributions

Despite acknowledged personhood variables, research has repeatedly demonstrated that the *strongest predictors* for the development of burnout

TABLE 3–2. Symptom overlap between early-stage burnout and clinical depression

Early-stage burnout	Major depression
Emotional depletion and exhaustion	Fatigue or loss of energy
Depersonalization (negative attitude toward patients and work responsibilities)	Lack of interest in pleasurable activities
Perceived lack of personal accomplishment	Feelings of personal worthlessness
Lack of motivation, especially for work-related tasks	Pervasive sad mood, manifesting across life domains
Irritation in response to job demands and lack of resources	Depressive episodes can have multiple triggers
Elevated risk of depression	Elevated risk of suicide

are actually *environmental*, such as work overload. Bakker and Demerouti's (2017) idea of job demands–resource theory reconceives burnout as developing from an imbalance between demands and resources. Problematic work demands in the medical and mental health professions include large caseloads or patient panels, lack of time for individual patient care, long hours, heavy call schedules, extensive administrative responsibilities, and diminished reimbursements. Both the emotional intensity of caring for patients and increased bureaucratic demands (e.g., electronic health records, paperwork such as prior authorizations and insurance forms), which take the mental health professional away from the more meaningful work of caring for patients, produce burnout (Shanafelt et al. 2017). As noted, emotional investment in the work is complex because overinvolvement predicts *both greater burnout and greater job satisfaction* for clinicians, suggesting a nuanced interaction between the two (Lee et al. 2011). Importantly, the perception of the work seems to predict the impact of work overload because emotional exhaustion (the first phase of burnout) is predicted only when the work is seen as a burden as opposed to a challenge.

Societal and Systemic Explanations

The development of burnout is closely entwined not only with the immediate work environment but also with the broader societal and cultural changes that have shaped our workplaces and workforces as a whole. Schaufeli et al. (2009) captured these historical shifts from a sociological perspective, emphasizing idealism and disillusionment of public service initiatives in the 1960s and 1970s, the cascading declines in the authority and prestige of the medical and mental health professions, and pervasive cultural shifts from community emphasis to individualism that erode social support. Industrialization and globalization have also contributed to a requirement to be "on" 24/7 because technology offers individuals electronic health records, email, and smartphones that allow people to never be untethered from work. Increasingly, demand outstrips supply of energy, personnel, equipment, and other resources. In turn, the values of individuals and the values of the organizations for whom they work drift further apart. The cumulative result is burnout.

Challenges to Preventing and Treating Burnout

Identifying and treating burnout are made more challenging by the historical practice of blaming the burned-out individual. With fully half of the medical profession experiencing some degree of burnout at any given point in time, this practice has clearly outlived its utility. Despite the pervasiveness of burnout, a lack of awareness of one's own burnout is common (Blackwelder et al. 2016). Even when the issue of awareness is overcome, the majority of clinicians who recognize their burnout continue to work even after the condition is recognized (Lee et al. 2011; Norcross 2005). Health care professionals also fail to confront burned-out colleagues or offer assistance for their burnout, and employees dramatically underutilize the organizational support services that are offered (Lee et al. 2011). Effectively reducing burnout in the medical workforce will likely require intervention at every level of the health care system.

Untreated Burnout and Mental Illness

Burnout is strongly correlated with mental health concerns, including increased rates of depression (Tennant 2001), substance abuse, and suicide (Dyrbye et al. 2008). In fact, some directional studies suggest that burnout is an active precursor to mental health issues, such as depression, and may be part of the underlying cause in some cases (Tennant 2001). Mental health clinicians are affected by psychiatric symptoms (e.g., anxiety, depression, substance abuse) at a higher frequency than the general population (Forbes et al. 2019). Mental health clinicians also have double the suicide rate (Center et al. 2003). With concerns about stigma, difficulties accepting help, and worries about how treatment may affect their ability to maintain professional licenses, clinicians are less likely to seek help than are individuals in the general population (Louie et al. 2007).

Depression

Although physicians appear to have rates of depression similar to those observed in the general population, medical students and residents are at higher risk for depression. In 2016, *JAMA* published a systematic review and meta-analysis that examined self-report data on the prevalence of depression or depressive symptoms in 167 cross-sectional studies of medical students in 43 countries (Rotenstein et al. 2016). The pooled prevalence of depression was 27.2%. Only 15.7% of those individuals screening positive for depression sought psychiatric treatment. Additionally, 11.1% of students surveyed by self-report measures in 24 cross-sectional studies reported suicidal ideation.

In 2010, another study indicated that female medical students were more likely than males to experience moderate to severe depression. Among both males and females, third- and fourth-year students demonstrated higher rates of suicidal ideation compared with students in the first 2 years (Schwenk et al. 2010). Even more concerning are data in the same study suggesting that students believe depression may cause them to be less respected by peers and may persuade faculty to perceive them as unable to handle their responsibilities. Students in the first 2 years of medical school were also more likely to believe that seeking help for depression would make them feel less intelligent.

Substance Abuse

Substance use disorders are estimated to affect between 10% and 15% of physicians, similar to the prevalence in the general population (Gastfriend 2005). The risk to patients when a physician is practicing while under the influence of substances is considerable, making the need for intervention perhaps even greater than for the general public. Fortunately, impaired physicians have increased access to comprehensive treatment through physician health programs, which aim to intervene early in the course of illness before patients are harmed. In fact, early voluntary participation in such programs can allow physicians to remain anonymous to state medical boards and the National Practitioner Data Bank. Physician health programs often include Alcoholics Anonymous participation, workplace surveillance, and random observed urine drug testing. Physicians are often highly motivated to participate in such programs, particularly because their license, livelihood, and professional identity are on the line (Gastfriend 2005). Recovery can be difficult, even for physicians; in one study, one in four monitored physicians relapsed at least once (Domino et al. 2005).

Suicide

Suicide is the only cause of mortality that is higher in physicians than in nonphysician peers (Albuquerque and Tulk 2019). In a study of nearly 8,000 surgeons, 15% of respondents had thought of suicide; 7% acknowledged suicidal ideation in the prior year; and more than one-third feared seeking care for ideation because of possible repercussions for their licensure or professional standing (Shanafelt et al. 2011). A six-school study of more than 2,000 medical students and residents found an overall suicidal ideation rate of 6% (Goebert et al. 2009). Trainees who identified as belonging to underrepresented minority groups were at highest risk, with 16% of Alaska Native, Native American, and Pacific Islander respondents and 13% of African American respondents reporting suicidal ideation. The relationship between burnout and suicide risk appears independent of symptoms of depression (Dyrbye et al. 2008).

Suicide risk among practicing physicians has long been recognized (Ross 1971). An American Foundation for Suicide Prevention planning group held a workshop in 2002 to develop a consensus statement concerning depression and suicide in physicians. At the time, they identified a number of barriers to identification and help seeking, including a culture of medicine that does not appear to prioritize physician mental health as well as licensing and hospital privileging that discriminate against those who have sought treatment for a mental health concern (Center et al. 2003). This risk is not unique to physicians. The American Psychological Association's Advisory Committee on Colleague Assistance initiated an ad hoc committee to investigate the prevalence and impact of psychologist suicide in 2011 (Kleespies et al. 2011). Eighteen percent of practitioners responding to a 2009 American Psychological Association Colleague Assistance and Wellness Survey acknowledged that they had experienced suicidal ideation (Kleespies et al. 2011).

Gender differences in completed suicide are also significant, with an aggregate suicide ratio compared with the general population of 1.41 for male physicians and 2.27 for female physicians (Schernhammer and Colditz 2004). As in the general population, firearms are the most common method for completed suicide in physicians, but higher numbers of physicians die by ingestion (potentially because they may have easier access to drugs) and blunt force trauma (Gold et al. 2013). For psychologists, findings are difficult to untangle, with conflicting reports and sometimes flawed studies. Proportionate mortality ratios indicate that white male and female psychologists have an elevated risk of suicide compared with the general population. Increased risk of suicide was not observed in black psychologists (National Occupational Mortality Surveillance System 2010).

Special Issues in Medical Training

Social and cultural dynamics surrounding physical health, mental health, and related concerns of suicidality and addiction in medical training were characterized in a novel study performed by one of us (L.W.R.). In this study of 1,027 students attending nine medical schools, 90% of medical students expressed a need for health care, with 54% acknowledging physical health issues and 46% acknowledging mental health care needs (Roberts et al. 2000, 2001). Of these students with health concerns, a majority (57%) did not seek "necessary care," and 48% encountered difficulties in obtaining care, such as being too busy to take time away from training (37%) and being too worried about the cost of care (28%). Confidentiality was of greatest concern among students in their clinical years of training. Sixty-three percent of students overall sought personal health care through informal "curbside consultation," with students in their clinical years using this approach for accessing health care services more heavily.

Many students in the study expressed significant concern about jeopardy to their academic status if their clinical supervising attendings or the dean's office learned about their health issues. The greatest concern was expressed for stigmatizing health issues, such as drug- or alcohol-related issues, HIV, depression, anxiety, eating disorders, and reproductive health issues (Roberts et al. 2001). Other issues, such as having cancer, relationship problems, or a serious infection, also triggered a sense of academic vulnerability. Students consistently expressed a robust preference for off-site care for stigmatizing or reproductive health needs. Women in this study more strongly expressed concern about potential stigma and potential negative grading or evaluations (Roberts et al. 2001, 2011b).

A subset of students ($n=955$) in the nine-school study responded to two vignettes that examined how students would handle a situation with a classmate who was actively suicidal and a student with observed erratic behavior and known alcohol and amphetamine use (Roberts et al. 2005). Medical student respondents said that they would "tell no one" about the classmate struggling with suicidality (45%) and about the student with addiction (53%), and only a small proportion (18% and 12%, respectively) would inform the dean's office about the issues in the two vignettes. Interestingly, the range of responses varied greatly by school, suggesting differing policies, practices, and cultures across institutions. For the suicidal classmate vignette, the range of response "tell no one" by school was 19%–70%, and for the student with addiction vignette, the range of response "tell no one" by school was 30%–70%.

In a follow-up study of residents ($N=155$) at one school (Moutier et al. 2009; Roberts and Kim 2015; Roberts et al. 2011a), a progression of health issues and similar care-seeking concerns were documented. In this study, 65% of residents reported a decline in their personal health over the course of residency, with worse decline among women respondents, and 16% of residents reported frequent health problems, with more frequent health issues reported by women respondents. Residents identified health care needs but avoided or delayed care "sometimes," reporting time constraints, privacy concerns, expense, and discomfort with the dual role as resident-patient as contributing reasons for avoiding or delaying necessary care. Informal "curbside" care was endorsed as a solution for access, with most residents indicating that they had sought curbside care in the past year as well as seeking care formally (80% and 70%, respectively). A large majority (90%) reported that their colleagues had asked for them to provide curbside care, and a significant minority of residents (28%) acknowledged that they had self-prescribed medications. The study also documented residents' concern about ostracism by peers and supervisors when residents needed to take time away from work for illness or health care appointments.

Accompanying the recognition of health issues of medical students and residents has been the painful acknowledgment of systemic mistreatment of physicians-in-training. The landmark study of students at the University of Colorado, published in 1990 (Silver and Glicken 1990), documented what had previously been depicted in fictional narratives, such as Samuel Shem's *The House of God.* A total of 431 medical students (83% response) participated in the Colorado study. Of these, 81% had experienced mistreatment or abuse by the end of their fourth year of medical school. The highest incidence was in the third year of training, with 20% of students experiencing at least five episodes of abusive treatment that was of "major importance and very upsetting."

In 2014, Fnais and colleagues published a comprehensive analysis of the prevalence of harassment, abuse, and discrimination among medical students and residents. Across studies, attending physicians, other health professionals, and, interestingly, patients engaged in negative behaviors such as harassment, abuse, and discrimination. The studies were heterogeneous in their methods, approaches, and measures. Nevertheless, these data suggest that the adverse influences on medical student and resident well-being are profound during medical training.

These findings, taken together, help to elucidate the stresses and patterns that emerge early in medical education. Physicians-in-training have made clear that seeking health care services, at least in the recent past, has been problematic because of many different potential obstacles (e.g., access, time, cost, stigma, academic jeopardy). Medical students, residents, and practicing physicians have indicated in multiple studies that they avoid necessary care and seek informal curbside consultation to obtain diagnostic studies or evaluations, prescriptions for medications, and other services (Roberts et al. 2000, 2005). Mistreatment of medical students and residents has been documented for many years, with harassment, discrimination, and abuse being far too commonly reported. For these reasons, Roberts has commented:

> Medical schools are entrusted with transforming bright and humanistic students into capable, compassionate physicians who will dedicate their lives to serving others. How best to fulfill this responsibility has emerged as a central concern of the medical profession. Research and self-honest observation over decades have revealed that many of the experiences of medical school may overwhelm and exhaust rather than inspire and instruct students. Indeed, contrary to the intent of medical educators, the experiences of medical training may damage the well-being and diminish the professionalism of many early career colleagues. (Roberts 2010, pp. 1231)

Positive Practices

The positive practices below relate to identifying early signs of burnout and finding appropriate support. They are applicable for professionals at any career stage.

1. Understand your own current level of burnout symptoms. Fill out the Stanford Professional Fulfillment Index (see Table 3–1). Are you surprised by any of the results?

2. Share experiences with colleagues and trusted friends. If experiencing symptoms of burnout, talk to someone about your feelings and seek support.
3. If a colleague comes to express symptoms of burnout, offer support. It can be helpful to acknowledge how common those symptoms are and also how they warrant additional intervention.
4. Educate yourself about relevant resources in the organization beforehand so you know where to turn if you or someone you work with needs additional help with symptoms of burnout or mental health challenges.

Conclusion

The pervasiveness of burnout among mental health professionals is a grave concern, especially given the associated risks to both clinicians and their patients. At every stage of professional development, access to individual confidential resources for combating burnout and treating mental health problems is critical. Strong social support in the workplace and a sense of inclusion and belonging can also help combat burnout. For instance, doctor-nurse relationships, colleague relationships, mentoring, peer support and supervision groups, and engagement in professional associations can all be protective factors across the professional life span (Norcross 2005). Finally, organizational and systemic interventions, such as inviting psychiatrists and psychologists into decision-making processes, streamlining case management, reducing administrative burden, and offering opportunities for professional development, are all organizational changes that are likely to be important in improving professional engagement and fulfillment (Lee et al. 2011).

Questions to Discuss With Colleagues and Mentors

—————o—————

- Does the three-part model of burnout—emotional exhaustion, cynicism, and reduced personal accomplishment—make sense to you?
- How does professional burnout differ from a mental disorder?
- Have you noticed that you are more likely to feel burned out with certain kinds of professional activities?
- What kinds of things do you do, personally and professionally, to fill your reservoir of resilience?

- What kinds of things can the workplace do to help minimize professional burnout and to foster resilience?

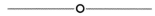

Recommended Resources

Eisenstein L: To fight burnout, organize. N Engl J Med 379:509–511, 2018

Gitlin M: Psychiatrist reactions to patient suicide: the clinician's role, in The American Psychiatric Publishing Textbook of Suicide Assessment and Management, 2nd edition. Edited by Simon RI, Hales RE. Arlington, VA, American Psychiatric Publishing, 2012

LoboPrabhu S, Summers RF, Moffic HS (eds): Combating Physician Burnout: A Guide for Psychiatrists. Washington, DC, American Psychiatric Association Publishing, 2020

Roberts LW: Clinician well-being and impairment, in A Clinical Guide to Psychiatric Ethics. Edited by Roberts LW. Arlington, VA, American Psychiatric Association Publishing, 2016, pp 223–236

Roberts LW, Trockel M (eds): The Art and Science of Physician Wellbeing. A Handbook for Physicians and Trainees. Cham, Switzerland, Springer, 2019

Rössler W: Burnout and disillusionment, in Leadership in Psychiatry. Edited by Bhugra D, Ruiz P, Gupta S. West Sussex, UK, Wiley, 2013, pp 199–205

Yellowlees P: Physician Suicide: Cases and Commentaries. Washington, DC, American Psychiatric Association Publishing, 2019

References

Albuquerque J, Tulk S: Physician suicide. CMAJ 191(18):E505, 2019 31061076

Bakker AB, Demerouti E: Job demands–resources theory: taking stock and looking forward. J Occup Health Psychol 22(3):273–285, 2017 27732008

Barnett JE, Baker EK, Elman NS, Schoener GR: In pursuit of wellness: the self-care imperative. Prof Psychol Res Pr 38(6):603–612, 2007

Blackwelder R, Watson KH, Freedy JR: Physician wellness across the professional spectrum. Prim Care 43(2):355–361, 2016 27262013

Bodenheimer T, Sinsky C: From triple to quadruple aim: care of the patient requires care of the provider. Ann Fam Med 12(6):573–576, 2014 25384822

Brazeau CM, Shanafelt T, Durning SJ, et al: Distress among matriculating medical students relative to the general population. Acad Med 89(11):1520–1525, 2014 25250752

Center C, Davis M, Detre T, et al: Confronting depression and suicide in physicians: a consensus statement. JAMA 289(23):3161–3166, 2003 12813122

Chaukos D, Chad-Friedman E, Mehta DH, et al: Risk and resilience factors associated with resident burnout. Acad Psychiatry 41(2):189–194, 2017 28028738

Domino KB, Hornbein TF, Polissar NL, et al: Risk factors for relapse in health care professionals with substance use disorders. JAMA 293(12):1453–1460, 2005 15784868

Dyrbye LN, Shanafelt TD: Physician burnout: a potential threat to successful health care reform. JAMA 305(19):2009–2010, 2011 21586718

Dyrbye LN, Thomas MR, Massie FS, et al: Burnout and suicidal ideation among U.S. medical students. Ann Intern Med 149(5):334–341, 2008 18765703

Fnais N, Soobiah C, Chen MH, et al: Harassment and discrimination in medical training: a systematic review and meta-analysis. Acad Med 89(5):817–827, 2014 24667512

Forbes MP, Jenkins K, Myers MF: Optimising the treatment of doctors with mental illness. Aust N Z J Psychiatry 53(2):106–108, 2019 30518249

Gastfriend DR: Physician substance abuse and recovery: what does it mean for physicians—and everyone else? JAMA 293(12):1513–1515, 2005 15784877

Goebert D, Thompson D, Takeshita J, et al: Depressive symptoms in medical students and residents: a multischool study. Acad Med 84(2):236–241, 2009 19174678

Gold KJ, Sen A, Schwenk TL: Details on suicide among US physicians: data from the National Violent Death Reporting System. Gen Hosp Psychiatry 35(1):45–49, 2013 23123101

Kahill S: Symptoms of professional burnout: a review of the empirical evidence. Can Psychol 29(3):284–297, 1988

Kleespies PM, Van Orden KA, Bongar B, et al: Psychologist suicide: incidence, impact, and suggestions for prevention, intervention, and postvention. Prof Psychol Res Pr 42(3):244–251, 2011 21731175

Kristensen TS, Borritz M, Villadsen E, Christensen KB: The Copenhagen Burnout Inventory: a new tool for the assessment of burnout. Work and Stress 19(3):192–207, 2005

Lee J, Lim N, Yang E, Lee SM: Antecedents and consequences of three dimensions of burnout in psychotherapists: a meta-analysis. Prof Psychol Res Pr 42(3):252–258, 2011

Louie A, Coverdale J, Roberts LW: Balancing the personal and the professional: should and can we teach this? Acad Psychiatry 31(2):129–132, 2007 17344452

MacKinnon M, Murray S: Reframing physician burnout as an organizational problem: a novel pragmatic approach to physician burnout. Acad Psychiatry 42(1):123–128, 2018 28247366

Maslach C, Goldberg J: Prevention of burnout: new perspectives. Appl Prev Psychol 7(1):63–74, 1998

Maslach C, Jackson SE: The measurement of experienced burnout. J Organ Behav 2(2):99–113, 1981

Maslach C, Leiter MP: Understanding the burnout experience: recent research and its implications for psychiatry. World Psychiatry 15(2):103–111, 2016 27265691

Moutier C, Cornette M, Lehrmann J, et al: When residents need health care: stigma of the patient role. Acad Psychiatry 33(6):431–441, 2009 19933883

National Occupational Mortality Surveillance System: Suicide in Psychologists. National Occupational Mortality Surveillance System (NOMS) Data (1984–1998). Atlanta, GA, Centers for Disease Control and Prevention, 2010.

Norcross JC: The psychotherapist's own psychotherapy: educating and developing psychologists. Am Psychol 60(8):840–850, 2005 16351423

Roberts LW: Understanding depression and distress among medical students. JAMA 304(11):1231–1233, 2010

Roberts LW, Kim JP: Informal health care practices of residents: "curbside" consultation and self-diagnosis and treatment. Acad Psychiatry 39(1):22–30, 2015 24923781

Roberts LW, Warner TD, Carter D, et al: Caring for medical students as patients: access to services and care-seeking practices of 1,027 students at nine medical schools. Collaborative Research Group on Medical Student Healthcare. Acad Med 75(3):272–277, 2000 10724317

Roberts LW, Warner TD, Lyketsos C, et al: Perceptions of academic vulnerability associated with personal illness: a study of 1,027 students at nine medical schools. Collaborative Research Group on Medical Student Health. Compr Psychiatry 42(1):1–15, 2001 11154710

Roberts LW, Warner TD, Rogers M, et al: Medical student illness and impairment: a vignette-based survey study involving 955 students at 9 medical schools. Collaborative Research Group on Medical Student Health Care. Compr Psychiatry 46(3):229–237, 2005 16021594

Roberts LW, Warner TD, Moutier C, et al: Are doctors who have been ill more compassionate? Attitudes of resident physicians regarding personal health issues and the expression of compassion in clinical care. Psychosomatics 52(4):367–374, 2011a 21777720

Roberts LW, Warner TD, Smithpeter M, et al: Medical students as patients: implications of their dual role as explored in a vignette-based survey study of 1027 medical students at nine medical schools. Compr Psychiatry 52(4):405–412, 2011b 21683176

Ross M: Suicide among physicians. Psychiatry Med 2(3):189–198, 1971 4948172

Rotenstein LS, Ramos MA, Torre M, et al: Prevalence of depression, depressive symptoms, and suicidal ideation among medical students: a systematic review and meta-analysis. JAMA 316(21):2214–2236, 2016 27923088

Schaufeli WB, Leiter MP, Maslach C: Burnout: 35 years of research and practice. Career Development International 14(3):204–220, 2009

Schernhammer ES, Colditz GA: Suicide rates among physicians: a quantitative and gender assessment (meta-analysis). Am J Psychiatry 161(12):2295–2302, 2004 15569903

Schwenk TL, Davis L, Wimsatt LA: Depression, stigma, and suicidal ideation in medical students. JAMA 304(11):1181–1190, 2010 20841531

Shanafelt TD, Noseworthy JH: Executive leadership and physician well-being: nine organizational strategies to promote engagement and prevent burnout. Mayo Clin Proc 92(1):129–146, 2017 27871627

Shanafelt TD, Sloan JA, Habermann TM: The well-being of physicians. Am J Med 114(6), 513–519, 2003 12727590

Shanafelt TD, Balch CM, Dyrbye L, et al: Special report: suicidal ideation among American surgeons. Arch Surg 146(1):54–62, 2011 21242446

Shanafelt TD, Boone S, Tan L, et al: Burnout and satisfaction with work-life balance among US physicians relative to the general US population. Arch Intern Med 172(18):1377–1385, 2012 22911330

Shanafelt TD, Hasan O, Dyrbye LN, et al: Changes in burnout and satisfaction with work-life balance in physicians and the general US working population between 2011 and 2014. Mayo Clin Proc 90(12):1600–1613, 2015 26653297

Shanafelt TD, Dyrbye LN, West CP: Addressing physician burnout: the way forward. JAMA 317(9):901–902, 2017 28196201

Silver HK, Glicken AD: Medical student abuse: incidence, severity, and significance. JAMA 263(4):527–532, 1990 2294324

Simionato GK, Simpson S: Personal risk factors associated with burnout among psychotherapists: a systematic review of the literature. J Clin Psychol 74(9):1431–1456, 2018 29574725

Tennant C: Work-related stress and depressive disorders. J Psychosom Res 51(5):697–704, 2001 11728512

Trockel M, Bohman B, Lesure E, et al: A brief instrument to assess both burnout and professional fulfillment in physicians: reliability and validity, including correlation with self-reported medical errors, in a sample of resident and practicing physicians. Acad Psychiatry 42(1):11–24, 2018 29196982

Vahey DC, Aiken LH, Sloane DM, et al: Nurse burnout and patient satisfaction. Med Care 42(2)(suppl):II57–II66, 2004 14734943

Wilson G, Larkin V, Redfern N, et al: Exploring the relationship between mentoring and doctors' health and wellbeing: a narrative review. J R Soc Med 110(5):188–197, 2017 28504073

World Health Organization: ICD-11 for Mortality and Morbidity Statistics, 2018. Available at: https://icd.who.int/browse11/l-m/en. Accessed December 13, 2019.

স

ॐ॰ॐ

CHAPTER 4

Approaches to Mental Health Care for Fellow Clinicians

Professionals providing mental health care are themselves vulnerable to mental health concerns. Physicians are affected by psychiatric symptoms, such as anxiety, depression, and substance abuse, at a higher frequency than the general population (Forbes et al. 2019). As a result, they have double the suicide rate (Center et al. 2003). Faced with concerns about stigma, difficulties accepting help, and worries about how treatment may affect their ability to maintain professional licenses, they are less likely to seek help than are individuals in the general population (Louie et al. 2007). These significant issues can also make mental health professionals more vulnerable to the negative long-term outcomes of inadequately treated mental illnesses. When treating colleagues, psychiatrists and psychologists have a responsibility to consider how to best reduce stigma and barriers to accessing care and how to optimize treatment effectiveness for fellow clinicians. In this chapter, we focus on the rewards and challenges of treating colleagues and offer recommendations for addressing the specific needs of the clinician-patient.

Unique Burdens of Clinician-Patients

The process of becoming a clinician and then practicing in the mental health field can contribute to the risk for mental health concerns. Medicine and mental health care can be extraordinarily gratifying professions, with patients and families allowing clinicians to be involved in personal

81

times of joy, pain, tragedy, healing, and heartbreak. It can also be challenging to tolerate uncertainty and to experience negative outcomes even when it feels as if everything has been done to try to prevent them.

Medicine is a demanding profession, requiring a certain amount of education, expense, and delayed gratification to achieve. The average physician has had 8 years of schooling after high school graduation, with 3–10 years of residency and fellowship training on top of that. Student loans in excess of $100,000 are not uncommon, and clinicians-in-training have worked long hours that may have made it difficult to stay connected to family, friends, and hobbies. After all of that time and money has been invested, not every graduate is happy with his or her career choice, yet there may be pressure to work in the chosen field in order to earn the salary needed to pay back student loans (Balch et al. 2009). Psychology graduate students fare little better, with 4–5 postcollege schooling years followed by internship, postdoctoral fellowship, and often lower prospects for financial compensation relative to peers with comparable years of schooling in other professions.

In addition to the challenges of the training years, practicing in the mental health field can be emotionally taxing. Many psychiatric patients have horrific histories that can actually cause secondary trauma to the treating clinician. Some patients attempt or even die from suicide. Patients, families, and physician colleagues in other specialties may have unrealistic expectations of what can be achieved in treatment. Unlike other areas of medicine, gains are most often measured in reduction and management of symptoms as opposed to "cures." Although many patients are grateful and appreciative of care, others may become angry when limits are placed on inappropriate behavior. They also may find it difficult to adhere to treatment recommendations or fail to make any sort of sustained behavior change, contributing to further burnout for treating clinicians.

All of these challenges may contribute to and exacerbate anxiety, depression, or other health conditions for the practicing clinician. As such, the assessment of a clinician-patient's presenting problems should include consideration of the contribution of his or her professional role. Professionals treating fellow clinicians may want to consider additionally discussing appropriate pragmatic supports, such as financial counseling, for clinician-patients. They may also want to normalize the stress of the profession and ensure that space is made for the clinician-patient to discuss fears of choosing the wrong profession or the desire to change fields.

The Clinician as a Patient

Physicians and other mental health clinicians are at once the same and uniquely different from any other patient. Psychiatrists and psychologists enjoy working with physician-patients. Physician-patients are generally very high functioning, verbal, intelligent, self-aware, and insightful about their interpersonal challenges (Norcross 2005). Primary care doctors report an increased emotional connection to their physician-patients (Stanton and Randal 2016). Camaraderie can result from a shared experience of training and experiencing similar pressures in personal and career development. Treating mental health professionals is a mixed blessing, however. Although there is an honor conferred in being designated the "doctor's doctor" or the "therapist's therapist," there is also increased pressure and unique demands in the role. For instance, physicians may have perfectionistic tendencies, may overinternalize work pressures, and may have trouble asking for help (Forbes et al. 2019). Several common issues faced by mental health professionals treating fellow clinicians are illustrated in the following vignette.

Vignette

As a newly licensed psychologist, Christy Baden was settling into her new job in an anxiety treatment clinic. One day, her boss pulled her aside and asked if he could talk to her about a potential case. Dr. Baden learned that a well-respected colleague was seeking treatment in the clinic. Her boss said he did not want to turn the prospective clinician-patient away because it would be difficult for her to find a therapist who would be covered by her insurance. Dr. Baden completed an evaluation and offered treatment because she was the only one with openings in her caseload and the only staff member who did not already know the patient. Even though Dr. Baden was well trained in the treatment of anxiety symptoms, she found herself intimidated by the prospect of treating a fellow clinician. When she started her intake, she skipped over questions and was unwilling to ask anything obvious. When it was time to provide treatment recommendations, she quickly outlined her recommended treatment plan but tried to avoid explaining in detail, for fear of insulting the well-informed patient. When the session ended, Dr. Baden could not stop obsessing over what she might have done wrong and whether her performance would negatively impact her professional reputation. Reflecting on the session later that evening, Dr. Baden realized she needed to seek additional consultation, likely outside of her workplace, in order to provide effective treatment for this patient.

It can be tempting to confuse the patient's motivations or experiences with one's own. Clinicians who work with psychiatrists and psychologists should be careful to seek out supervision around boundaries when caring for patients. Clinicians also report greater self-consciousness and evaluative fears when treating colleagues (Forbes et al. 2019). Their concerns are not without merit because physician-patients acknowledge evaluating the competence and decisiveness of their clinicians (Stanton and Randal 2016). Psychiatrists and psychologists are inherently more savvy consumers and thus typically are selective in choosing mental health professionals, preferring well-respected senior clinicians (Norcross 2005; Stanton and Randal 2016). Recommendations are made in this chapter not only for attuning to the needs of the clinician-patient but also for considering the unique impacts on the treating clinician.

Experience of the Treating Clinician

Collectively, the research on treating doctors and other mental health professionals reflects that clinicians experience a strong desire to help as well as a desire to impress. Along with the desire to impress comes a common feeling of insecurity about knowledge or skills and fears of criticism from the wider medical community if an adverse outcome occurs (Forbes et al. 2019; Norcross 2005; Stanton and Randal 2016). The result is often heightened self-monitoring overall.

Clinicians additionally reported greater awareness than usual that they could easily be the patient as well as the physician, leading to increased empathy and/or increased self-consciousness and urge to distance (Norcross 2005; Stanton and Randal 2016). Collegiality made it harder to bring up issues, and, often, there was an early impression of cooperation on the part of the clinician-patient that turned out to be the patient's avoidance and desire to not be difficult. In turn, this avoidance ultimately led to disengagement. Having seniority in the field, prior experience treating patients who were physicians or other mental health practitioners, and a personal history of therapy themselves helped mitigate these challenges.

Access to Care: Stigma and the Culture of Physician Invulnerability

Physicians are steeped in a culture of invulnerability (Baker and Sen 2016). Although there are recent positive shifts toward a greater culture of wellness, historically, messages have been given to physicians-in-training and other clinician trainees that a competent health professional is a stoic one. There is little to no space for vulnerability, and self-sacrifice as opposed to self-care has been historically valued and rewarded (Baker and Sen 2016; Forbes et al. 2019). Some mental health professionals suggest that these issues lead doctors to develop a stance of omnipotence and detachment (Forbes et al. 2019). An "us versus them" mentality results, in which similarities between patients and doctors—a so-called *common humanity*—are minimized. The result is a heightening of stigma around seeking treatment and unhelpful shame and self-blame for being in the patient role (Forbes et al. 2019).

This patient-clinician separation can be further reinforced by the "medical illness" lens sometimes used in psychiatry. Although therapeutic traditions, such as psychology, social work, and nursing, have increasingly moved toward a culture of wellness (e.g., emphasizing acceptance, compassion, and growth enhancement aspects of psychotherapy), there is clearly room for continued progress. Stigmatizing language, such as references to "mentally ill" clinicians, can be expected to naturally deepen the "doctor versus patient" divide and underscore the sense of stigma around seeking treatment. Physicians treated for common struggles, such as depression, anxiety, stress, and burnout, may benefit from a therapeutic approach steeped in contemporary therapeutic acceptance and self-compassion theory as opposed to a heavily medicalized psychopathology lens. As illustrated in the following vignette, it can be quite difficult for clinicians to face their own vulnerability.

Vignette

Jared Xu had been working on the inpatient psychiatry unit for about a year. He became discouraged observing patients return to the unit after discharge, sometimes with symptoms worse than those experienced during their first hospitalizations. One day, while explaining the diagnostic criteria for a major depressive episode to a trainee, Dr. Xu admitted to himself that he, too, was experiencing serious symptoms of depression. He was well aware that most of the patients he treated on a daily basis were much worse than he was, and he tried to push the thoughts out of his mind. He told himself, "look around you, you have no excuse to feel so bad" and "get over yourself." Over time, his depression symptoms progressed until one of his colleagues noticed the change and confronted him about seeking treatment.

In addition to feelings of shame and self-consciousness about seeking treatment and reticence to be in the patient role, mental health professionals report fears that their concerns are trivial. They feel that they are wasting the clinician's time or that their professional license could be jeopardized by seeking treatment (Stanton and Randal 2016). Directly normalizing clinicians seeking treatment and offering reassurance as to the importance of their care are likely to be beneficial.

The personality traits of physicians can impact care. Although every physician is different, traits of perfectionism and a tendency toward obsessiveness are common in the field. These characteristics are advantageous during schooling and in medical careers, allowing mental health professionals to excel academically and reduce errors (Stanton and Randal 2016). However, they also tend to work against openness, flexibility, and relinquishing a control agenda in therapy, which are important for optimizing greater patient well-being.

Physicians need to be able to seek care separately from their own systems, where they will not encounter their patients and colleagues (Figure 4–1). When possible, it is important to avoid dual relationships. It helps to know that billing will be processed by people with whom they do not directly work, for example. They also need to be able to fill prescriptions comfortably, without the worry that pharmacy staff members will recognize their name or comment on their status as a patient. Physicians are often concerned about taking time away from work for treatment, as some worry that people will question their commitment to the job. In addition, they may have to manage the consequences of a psychiatric diagnosis on their record when it comes to buying life or disability insurance or when applying for professional licensure.

Changing Cultures of Wellness

In training, many residents and graduate students seek psychotherapy as a way to hold themselves accountable with boundaries, to learn more about therapy by experiencing it in the patient role, and to explore their own motivations and behaviors and the ways that they may impact clinical work (Norcross 2005). In contrast to historical messages about the invulnerability of clinicians, entering psychotherapy during training is often viewed as an accepted and even desirable part of the process of becoming a clinician. Some programs offer free or reduced-fee sessions to trainees. Once training is complete, fewer attending physicians are open to continuing in ongoing psychotherapy. One way to begin to reverse this pattern is by talking more openly about care.

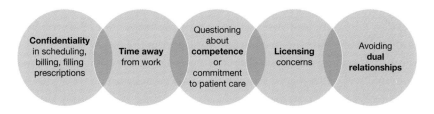

FIGURE 4–1. Physician concerns regarding accessing mental health care.

Source. Image created by Jennifer L. Derenne and Grace W. Gengoux.

Improving Access to Care: Transparency and Direct Communication

The culture of medicine has historically promoted suppression of emotion, denial of vulnerability, exacting standards, and impeccable professionalism. This indoctrination has been dubbed a "bullying culture" (Stanton and Randal 2016) and can dissuade physician-patients from speaking openly about their concerns in training. Psychiatrist-patients in Stanton and Randal's study reported that they valued openness and honesty, yet these ideas conflicted with both their training culture and their desire to be a "good patient" (i.e., not burden their doctor). Additionally, there was a tendency to report symptoms in an intellectualized manner, with much greater difficulty speaking of emotional experience or "from the heart" to "tell their story."

Colleagues treating other physicians or mental health professionals can learn valuable lessons from these reports. First, explicitly setting a framework for open communication is vital. Mental health professionals can empathize with the clinician-patient regarding how the culture works against seeking help and highlight how doing so is a sign of strength. They can assure the clinician-patient that his or her emotions can be freely expressed and explain that there is a willingness to truly listen without needing to feel protected from burdens or an expectation of being an "easy patient." Mental health professionals should explicitly redefine being a "good patient" as being open, honest, and non-self-censoring and speaking from the heart without editorializing.

Stanton and Randal (2016) found that clinician-patients tended not to openly ask for needs to be met, regardless of whether the need was for more or less intervention from their doctors. Rather, clinician-patients reported distancing themselves, struggling to form an alliance with the treating clinician, and disengaging from the treatment (Stanton and Randal 2016). Again, open communication from the outset is an obvious solution. Treating clinicians should inquire about the clinician-patient's preferred style with regard to giving advice and accommodate or discuss collaboratively the potential drawbacks of shifting style. Simply sharing information with a patient about what leads physicians to drop out of treatment may help prevent it.

Informal Consultation

Given the high levels of stigma associated with seeking care and a tendency for clinicians to self-treat (Balon 2007) or consult friends and family instead (Baker and Sen 2016), clinicians may be more likely to seek informal consultation from colleagues as opposed to formal treatment. Mentorship and peer consultation is an extremely helpful resource, not only for professional development but also for support around work stress, burnout prevention, and managing challenging patients and personal reactions (Wilson et al. 2017). Informal consultation should not replace formal treatment when it is needed. When physicians consult informally with colleagues about health concerns, rather than encouraging then to make an appointment, Forbess and colleagues (2019) cite lack of role clarity, insufficient assessment, and inadequate documentation as several of the risks and drawbacks associated with providing curbside consultation to colleagues around their own health concerns.

For confidentiality concerns, any professional consultation made by treating clinicians with mentors, consultants, or peer professionals should occur outside the patient's practice network or place of work. Not discussing the treatment with colleagues of the clinician-patient, even informally, is also an important consideration. Doing so would cause discomfort (Stanton and Randal 2016) and may call into question how seriously boundaries and confidentiality are handled.

Pragmatic Accommodations

After stigma and confidentiality, time and scheduling challenges top a clinician's list of barriers to care (Baker and Sen 2016). Trainees, in particular, typically have grueling schedules that do not easily permit appointments during traditional business hours. Offering after-hours or other nontraditional appointment types, such as telehealth visits or weekend appointments, or showing flexibility week to week for ongoing therapy care rather than requiring a set time can increase accessibility for clinician-patients. Prioritizing and expediting services are also encouraged, although health professionals should be thoughtful about the clinical appropriateness of flex schedules on a case-by-case basis. For psychotherapy, for instance, failure to establish regular appointments can be detrimental to alliance, momentum, and gold standard care that reflects empirically based protocols. Clinicians who frequently treat VIP patients for whom standard hours, wait times, or treatment approaches are made flexible or other requests are accommodated are all too familiar with the cliché that VIP patients get the worst care because of the inherent loss of the treatment frame and how far treatment can stray from what is known from research. Flexibility without boundary crossing or loss of best practices is optimal. Table 4–1 outlines strategies clinicians can use to encourage colleagues to access mental health care when appropriate.

The Clinician-Patient: Three Case Discussions

The following three case examples illustrate common challenges in providing mental health care to fellow clinicians and recommended strategies that can be used to effectively address issues that often arise. Research finds that clinician-patients engage in high levels of selective disclosure, possibly out of denial or to avoid an unwanted diagnosis (Forbes et al. 2019). First and foremost, treating clinicians should offer a warm, nonjudgmental stance to help combat stigma. Second, openness and transparency in discussing how the clinician-patient is experiencing care may help prevent alliance rupture and premature termination. Mental health professionals should check in regularly about the clinician-patient's experience. Physicians and other mental health professionals report strong desires to be a "good patient," which can lead to reluctance to voice disagreement about the treatment plan, withdrawal from the therapeutic relationship, and, ultimately, disengagement with treatment (Stanton and Randal 2016).

Clinician-patients vary in the extent to which they value a collaborative, democratic process as opposed to wanting the treating physician to serve as the expert and the authority on a diagnosis and treatment plan (Stanton and Randal 2016). Finding a balance between lay language and medical jargon is also key because the former risks being insulting and the latter risks affecting a distanced, intellectual discussion. With appropriate consent, some clinicians have encouraged the practice of obtain-

---

TABLE 4–1. Ways clinicians can encourage colleagues to access appropriate mental health care

---

- Praise efforts at improving physician well-being as being good for patient outcomes and relationships with family and friends.
- Explicitly encourage physician-patients to be honest and open and to resist the urge to be a "good patient."
- Without blurring boundaries, find ways to offer physicians flexibility with scheduling to avoid missed or late appointments.
- Offer mental health services and pharmacies at facilities separate from the workplace, with confidential scheduling and billing practices.
- Review state-specific licensing questions to determine whether seeking mental health care will truly impact future licensing.

---

ing a clinician-patient's old medical records and collateral information from family and friends as an avenue to combat physician denial and selective sharing of history (Forbes et al. 2019). Mental health professionals should consider the costs and benefits on a case-by-case basis and in collaboration with the clinician-patient.

The cases below illustrate the unique confidentiality, scheduling, and billing concerns that are prevalent for clinician-patients, as well as the considerations that often go into selection of a potential health professional. The cases also illustrate the challenge clinicians face in deciding how much to modify their traditional care practices to accommodate a clinician-patient.

Together, these three case studies highlight how effective treatment of fellow clinicians may require adjustments to aspects of usual practice. At the same time, clinicians treating colleagues have to be vigilant and obtain their own supervision or consultation as necessary to ensure that any accommodations do not inappropriately violate professional boundaries or weaken the effectiveness of the care provided. A number of helpful tips for treating colleagues are summarized in Table 4–2. Following these guidelines can help mental health professionals maintain balance between the flexibility necessary to accommodate the clinician-patient's unique needs and the ability to continue to deliver high-quality care.

Case Example 1

Jody Waters is a general child and adolescent psychiatrist who has been in practice for 5 years. Although she used to feel appreciated by her pa-

---

TABLE 4–2. Tips for treating colleagues

- Keep in mind that many physicians hold themselves to high standards and may need to work on allowing themselves the flexibility to ask for help to prioritize their health and well-being.
- Normalize and validate help seeking as good self-care.
- Acknowledge the challenges of seeking care, particularly during training, given stigma and historical messaging in the medical and mental health fields about invulnerability.
- Because physicians worry about stigma, especially focused around others' perceptions of their job performance, it is important for them to feel that they have access to confidential mental health care in a private setting by clinicians who do not work regularly in their home system. Billing for these services should not be processed by their own staff.
- Many physicians are reluctant to seek mental health care for fear that it will cause problems with their medical licensure, so it is important to be aware of the regulations for the state where the physician is licensed. Some states ask whether the applicant has been in mental health treatment or has taken psychotropic medications, whereas others are interested in whether the applicant has any health conditions that prevent him or her from practicing medicine safely.
- Do not assume your patient has expertise in a particular diagnosis or treatment approach just because he or she is a physician or psychologist. Recommend resources and reading materials applicable to the individual's condition, in case your patient wants to learn more. While maintaining a respectful, collaborative approach, ask if the patient would appreciate psychoeducation just as you would with any other patient and check for understanding.
- Balance medical jargon with lay language to optimize being respectful of the clinician's knowledge without allowing the clinician-patient to become distant and to intellectualize his or her own experience.
- Be sensitive to the unique schedule demands of mental health professionals and be flexible where possible in accommodating after-hours appointments. Consider offering telehealth appointments where possible. It is important that those who work with clinician-patients examine self-motivations and boundaries around making changes to their usual practice. Balance flexibility with careful monitoring of unhelpful overaccommodation, such as ignoring repeated late arrivals, cancellations, or no-shows, because this can interfere with optimal treatment.
- Ask directly about the clinician-patient's experience of treatment and check in regularly.

TABLE 4–2.   Tips for treating colleagues *(continued)*

- Do not assume that the absence of expressed concerns and the appearance of cooperation necessarily mean a strong alliance. Clinician-patients tend to want to be "good patients" and not make demands, express dissent, or otherwise "burden" their treating clinician.
- If consultation with another clinician is needed to inform care, confirm that this person is outside the patient's professional network to maintain strict confidentiality.
- Take a humanizing stance that emphasizes growth and common experience over pathology and illness.
- Offer assurance that you can handle anything the clinician-patient has to share. Express that you are unconcerned about being burdened and emphasize hearing the clinician-patient's story as opposed to merely noting his or her symptoms.

---

tients and their families, she has been feeling burned out lately and has questioned her career choice. Despite her best efforts, her patients do not improve as quickly as everyone would like. She receives frequent calls from parents and teachers requesting that she change medications to better target her patients' behavioral issues. At the same time, she worries that medication management is really only a small part of the overall treatment plan and that the majority of these children are struggling because of chaotic, inconsistent home environments and parenting challenges. She really enjoys doing psychotherapy with her patients and their families, and it was the main reason she chose child psychiatry over a career in pediatrics. However, she has been discouraged from providing psychotherapy because there are a limited number of child psychiatrists in her area. Therefore, her health care system prefers that she provide psychopharmacology consultations and follow-ups and that psychotherapy be conducted by nonprescribing colleagues in her department. Dr. Waters has significant financial incentive to transition to a practice focused solely on medication management; she finds it easier to surpass her billing targets for bonus earnings when she is seeing three to four medication follow-up visits per hour compared with one psychotherapy patient.

Dr. Waters is also feeling stressed in her personal life. She married during her fellowship training and has two young children. Her spouse also works full time, and she shoulders much of the burden of cooking, cleaning, and childrearing within their household. She resents her partner because she feels the division of labor is unequal and unfair. She worries about the financial and emotional ramifications of ending the marriage, especially because their children are young.

Dr. Waters does not feel that she meets criteria for a mood or anxiety disorder, but she does feel that she could use the support of a psychotherapist to help her deal with work and home life challenges. Still, she is cautious with her savings in the event of a marriage separation, and money is tight. She cannot afford the out-of-pocket costs associated with a private practice therapist, but the only psychotherapists covered by her insurance plan are within her own department.

Understandably, Dr. Waters is worried about confidentiality. She wants to avoid a dual relationship with a therapist in her own office and also does not want billing from her personal mental health sessions to be processed by staff with whom she works on a professional level. She is afraid that she will be seen as "weak" or not competent at her job. She also worries that therapy will affect her medical license. Her strong preference is to work with an M.D. psychiatrist who "understands the pressure and has had similar experiences with training and career development."

After an annual review in which she was given feedback that staff thought she was moody and difficult to work with, Dr. Waters sought consultation with a peer mentor. She received an email about the peer mentoring as part of a new feature of a physician wellness program and was reassured by the fact that no records were kept of the contact or the content of the meetings. In their discussion, she learned that the institution had identified therapists in the community who were not affiliated with their system for precisely this purpose and that mental health billing for physician-patients was conducted off-site as well.

Dr. Waters used her health insurance to see a clinician with whom she felt comfortable, without fear that she would be stigmatized for seeking mental health care. She also learned about the nuances of the language her state medical board used to ask about physician impairment and was relieved to see that the question asked whether the applicant has had any medical or mental health problems that currently impact the ability to provide care, rather than asking blanket questions about having ever sought mental health treatment.

This case highlights a number of common issues. Dr. Waters is struggling with significant challenges in both her personal and her professional life but is hesitant to make an appointment because of confidentiality concerns and the potential licensing and career implications of seeking formal care. The peer mentor feature of her institution's physician wellness program offers her the ability to consult confidentially with a peer who does not keep session records and is able to give her up-to-date and clear advice about how best to navigate the system so that her own mental health needs are being adequately addressed.

Case Example 2

Mark Jones graduated from general psychiatry residency last year and has been adjusting to his new academic position working on an inpatient psychiatric unit. He has a history of classic bipolar disorder, with his first manic episode occurring in his senior year of undergraduate education. He has been mood stabilized on lithium since then, with a couple of mild depressive episodes that resolved quickly with adjustments to his psychotropic medication regimen. As a trainee, he had a number of different clinical rotations and felt able to find holes in his schedule that allowed him to "sneak away" to keep up with his follow-up psychiatry visits.

With the transition to an attending physician role and having a position consolidated in one place, Dr. Jones' schedule was much more predictable but also busier. He now must see double the number of patients he had seen as a resident physician. The staff, trainees, and his colleagues expect him to be available on the inpatient unit most of the time. Dr. Jones struggles to prioritize his medical appointments. He holds himself to high standards and worries that he is not meeting expectations if he takes time away during the workday.

While working with a very high functioning young professional who was admitted to the inpatient unit in a manic state due to a stressful work environment and lack of sleep, Dr. Jones realizes he should prioritize his own health to avoid a relapse. His personal psychiatrist is understanding of time and schedule constraints and blocks an appointment in his schedule so that he can reliably see Dr. Jones once per month. Dr. Jones feels comfortable asking a colleague to cover for him in the event that he is not able to get back to the unit on time for rounds, choosing to tell her that he needs to attend regular medical visits as part of his treatment for a chronic medical condition. On days when he is a little late arriving in the morning, he stays later in the evening to make up the time.

Dr. Jones' situation illustrates the very common predicament that physician-patients find themselves struggling to manage. He is conscientious and holds himself to high standards and feels guilty about not being present and available at every moment. Unfortunately, this misguided sense of responsibility is preventing him from taking the best possible care of himself, and he may in fact be unintentionally putting his patients at risk in the event that he experiences a mental health crisis that could impair his clinical abilities or force a substantial medical leave. He is ultimately able to reframe his thinking about the situation, recognizing that shifting his schedule slightly and relying on colleagues for help will possibly prevent future decompensation.

The psychiatrist who is treating Dr. Jones understands the practical issues with taking time away from a busy practice and is willing to offer him special appointment times. However, the psychiatrist will need ongoing reflection to prevent boundary violations that can arise from over-identifying with a patient.

Case Example 3

Sally Rivera, a mid-career psychiatrist in private practice, is approached by psychiatrist Dr. Chris Stanton for treatment of his depression. Dr. Stanton arrives 20 minutes late to his first session. Dr. Rivera greets him warmly and expresses empathy for Dr. Stanton's busy university schedule. She offers that today's schedule allows her to run a bit over, so they can still complete a full intake, but notes that typically she normally does not have much flexibility in her afternoons. She suggests that perhaps they talk later about alternative appointment times or other strategies that might help make attendance manageable for Dr. Stanton.

As they begin the intake, Dr. Rivera finds herself feeling uncharacteristically nervous and more acutely aware than usual of the language she selects. She observes Dr. Stanton looking around her office and taking in her diplomas and wonders what assumptions he might be making. She wants to be helpful to Dr. Stanton and put him at ease and is also mindful that she equally wishes to treat him as ordinarily as possible. Dr. Stanton quickly runs through his list of symptoms, making the diagnosis of depression for her and noting that his symptoms are "pretty mild." He says that he wishes to get ahead of any potential issues because depression does run in his family.

Dr. Rivera uses warmth and humor to joke with Dr. Stanton that he has done her work for her and gently explains that although she agrees depression sounds like it fits the symptom list, she would very much like to get to know him better and hear his story fully. She wonders aloud what his days are like personally and professionally, how the struggle with his mood is impacting his experience day to day, and how he came to the decision to come in for treatment. She additionally shares that she is glad that he did. From her perspective, she says, it shows a great deal of fortitude on his part because clinicians often avoid seeking treatment, to their detriment.

Dr. Stanton begins to share more about what he is experiencing, and the intake hour passes quickly. At the close of the session, Dr. Rivera shares her conceptualization and several treatment options with Dr. Stanton and asks how they sound to him. She invites his feedback on how he hopes their work together might proceed, both in terms of interest in therapy versus medication or a combined approach and in terms of the relationship fit. She shares her general style of working and welcomes Dr. Stanton's open and honest feedback about how the sessions will fit his needs. They agree to begin with a round of psychotherapy given the mild nature of Dr. Stanton's symptoms and identify a new early morning appointment time before he begins his typical clinic days.

Dr. Rivera came highly recommended to Dr. Stanton by a colleague, and he selected her because she is outside his professional network, has a strong background in evidence-based medicine, and is known for her warmth and expertise. He sought the referral some months ago, but work became extra busy and his teenage children needed additional support with academics, so he put the referral to the side. He almost canceled the appointment after a hectic day and the notion that maybe things were getting better anyway but decided at the last minute to attend. He is appreciative when Dr. Rivera acknowledges understanding about his schedule and works with him to find an optimal time. He had not realized he was quite so tardy until she said something. Dr. Stanton recognizes his ambivalence is partly to blame. Feeling reassured about the more optimal appointment time and Dr. Rivera's thoughtfulness in accommodating him, he hopes this will be a short-term process because she surely has patients in more need of her services.

Dr. Stanton is a practicing psychiatrist struggling with depression who seeks treatment with Dr. Rivera. This case discussion highlights the experience on both sides of the professional clinician-patient relationship and points to ways that mental health professionals can optimize treatment for their clinician-patients, neither shying away from asking important information nor failing to acknowledge the specialized needs of the clinician-patient. By talking openly and directly about the therapeutic relationship with someone in the field and soliciting feedback, Dr. Rivera put Dr. Stanton at ease, engaging him in the treatment planning and decreasing the likelihood that he would drop out of care. She also explicitly gave him permission to not play the "good patient" role and invited his sharing more openly and vulnerably. Finally, she briefly named the stigma that prevents some mental health professionals from seeking treatment and directly stated that she saw seeking support as a strength and a step toward healthy self-care.

Positive Practices

1. If you currently treat physicians or other mental health professionals in your practice, reflect on the extent to which you have had direct and open dialogue about their experience in your care. Did you bring up a discussion about their experience in your care or did the patient? How early in care? If you have not brought it up, consider doing so. Discuss the issues raised in this chapter with your clinician-patient and invite his or her reflection at a subsequent appointment, looking for space to discuss stigma, avoided content, preferred style, and feelings about treatment overall.
2. In addition to seeking information about the clinician-patient's experience, self-reflect on your own. If you are treating a fellow clini-

cian, take a moment to reflect on your personal experience of your work together. Are you feeling anxious or self-conscious? Do you find yourself practicing differently than you typically do? Do these changes feel comfortable and helpful to you both or do any feel uncomfortable or make you uneasy? Consider whether your patient's status as a clinician-patient is increasing or decreasing your use of peer consultation. If you are not currently consulting about your clinician-patient(s), consider with whom you would consult should you need to do so. This may require further consideration because your usual mentors may not be appropriate fits if they are within the same work setting of the clinician-patient.

3. Reflect on the systems in which you are embedded and particularly any areas where you might be in a leadership role. What policies are in place at your organization that support or deter employees from seeking mental health care? What unwritten rules about health care use by clinicians exist in the culture of your organization that are conveyed via modeling or attitude? What are two actions you might do this week to contribute to a movement toward a more positive culture? These steps could include inquiring about the policies, talking with coworkers about the culture of mental health use by employees, sharing concepts from this chapter at a work meeting, voicing support and encouragement of colleagues, or seeking care yourself (see Chapter 13, "Psychiatric Care and Psychotherapy").

Conclusion

Treating a physician or other mental health professional requires compassion, understanding, and expertise. Clinicians face all of the same mental health challenges and risks for psychiatric conditions prevalent in the general population. In addition, providing mental health care can be taxing, making psychiatrists and psychologists particularly vulnerable to burnout. A range of psychological supports, including psychotherapy, may be helpful to clinicians at different points in their professional work. Clinicians treating fellow psychiatrists or psychologists face the challenge of accommodating the unique needs of their colleagues while also maintaining sufficient treatment integrity for their interventions to work. Effective care for clinician-patients requires acknowledgment of major barriers to seeking care and creating flexible solutions to make accessing care more practical and confidential.

Questions to Discuss With Colleagues and Mentors

———————o———————

- What have been your own experiences treating colleagues? Do you have any advice to share regarding practice parameters for this sensitive work?
- When working with patient-colleagues, how can I make sure to engage in appropriate self-reflection and consultation? What do you suggest if I find that I have deviated from my typical practice?
- What recommendations do you have for obtaining consultation outside my usual network if my patient-colleague is known to many people in my professional network?

———————o———————

Recommended Resources

Accreditation Council for Graduate Medical Education: Improving physician well-being, restoring meaning in medicine. Chicago, IL, Accreditation Council for Graduate Medical Education. Available at: https://www.acgme.org/What-We-Do/Initiatives/Physician-Well-Being. Accessed December 13, 2019.

American Psychiatric Association: Well-being and burnout: take charge of your well-being. Washington, DC, American Psychiatric Association, 2019. Available at: www.psychiatry.org/psychiatrists/practice/wellbeing-and-burnout. Accessed December 13, 2019.

Forbes MP, Jenkins K, Myers MF: Optimising the treatment of doctors with mental illness. Austr N Z J Psychiatry 53(2):106–108, 2019

Houpt JL, Gilkey RW, Ehringhaus SH: Learning to Lead in the Academic Medical Center: A Practical Guide, New York, Springer, 2015

Ingelfinger FJ: Arrogance. N Engl J Med 303(26):1507–1511, 1980

Kansagra S: Everything I Learned in Medical School Besides All the Book Stuff. Author, 2011

King NMP, Strauss RP, Churchill LR, et al: The Social Medicine Reader, Volume 1. Durham, NC, Duke University Press, 2005

Lane LW, Lane G, Schiedermayer DL, et al: Caring for medical students as patients. Arch Intern Med 150(11): 2249–2253, 1990

Myers MF, Gabbard GO: Physician as Patient. Washington, DC, American Psychiatric Publishing, 2008

National Academy of Medicine: Action collaborative on clinician well-being and resilience. Washington, DC, National Academy of Medicine,

2019. Available at: https://nam.edu/initiatives/clinician-resilience-and-well-being. Accessed December 13, 2019.

Stanton J, Randal P: Developing a psychiatrist-patient relationship when both people are doctors: a qualitative study. BMJ Open 6(5):e010216, 2016

Starr P: The Social Transformation of American Medicine. New York, Basic Books, 1982

References

Baker K, Sen S: Healing medicine's future: prioritizing physician trainee mental health. AMA J Ethics 18(6):604–613, 2016 27322994

Balch CM, Freischlag JA, Shanafelt TD: Stress and burnout among surgeons: understanding and managing the syndrome and avoiding the adverse consequences. Arch Surg 144(4):371–376, 2009 19380652

Balon R: Psychiatrist attitudes toward self-treatment of their own depression. Psychother Psychosom 76(5):306–310, 2007, 17700051

Center C, Davis M, Detre T, et al: Confronting depression and suicide in physicians: a consensus statement. JAMA 289(23):3161–3166, 2003 12813122

Forbes MP, Jenkins K, Myers MF: Optimising the treatment of doctors with mental illness. Austr N Z J Psychiatry, 53(2):106–108 2019 30518249

Louie A, Coverdale J, Roberts LW: Balancing the personal and the professional: should and can we teach this? Acad Psychiatry 31(2):129–132, 2007 17344452

Norcross JC: The psychotherapist's own psychotherapy: educating and developing psychologists. Am Psychol 60(8):840–850, 2005 16351423

Stanton J, Randal P: Developing a psychiatrist-patient relationship when both people are doctors: a qualitative study. BMJ Open 6(5):e010216, 2016 27207623

Wilson G, Larkin V, Redfern N, et al: Exploring the relationship between mentoring and doctors' health and wellbeing: a narrative review. J R Soc Med 110(5):188–197, 2017 28504073

CHAPTER 5

Special Challenges for Clinicians-in-Training

The training period is a time of great potential but also a time of significant vulnerability. Students in the mental health professions may feel both excited about having chosen a career with tremendous potential for societal impact and nervous about the enormous responsibility of caring for people who are truly suffering. The Herman cartoon (Figure 5–1) captures the absurdity of abruptly transitioning from student to doctor. Given the vulnerable position of psychiatry and psychology students and the potential long-term effects of interventions to support these trainees, their well-being deserves special consideration. In this chapter, we discuss both professional and personal stressors that affect many preservice mental health professionals and potential supports to help enhance well-being during the training years and beyond.

Protecting the well-being and career longevity of existing and future mental health professionals is critical to the future of the health care industry. Current projections suggest that the United States will face a shortage of physicians in the near future. Medical school enrollment has consistently increased over the years, but estimates suggest that one-third of physicians will retire in the next decade, leading to shortages in primary care as well as specialty physicians necessary to care for a growing and aging population (Salsberg and Grover 2006).

Medical trainees—namely, students, residents, and fellows—are at particular risk of developing mental health difficulties and may have an even greater challenge accessing appropriate care compared with attending physicians. Trainees who are from underrepresented minorities or who are living with preexisting health conditions are at highest risk (Roberts 2010). Surveys of trainees in psychology doctoral programs

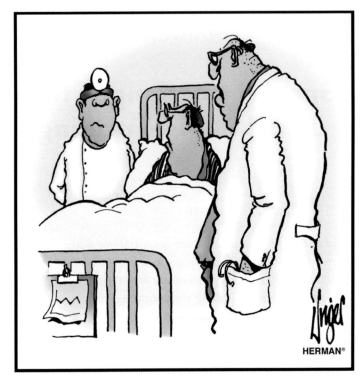

"You've got to start sometime. Why don't you operate on this one?"

FIGURE 5–1.   How it all begins.

Source.   HERMAN © 1998 LaughingStock International Inc. Reprinted by permission of ANDREWSMCMEEL SYNDICATION for UFS. All rights reserved.

and internships also indicate that mental health concerns can lead to problems with clinical deficiency, interpersonal issues, supervision, and physical illness (Huprich and Rudd 2004). Many trainees neglect self-care in order to optimize performance at work. Trainees who are being evaluated may worry that a lackluster assessment might jeopardize their chances for a desirable residency or fellowship position.

Achievement-Oriented Character Traits and the Culture of Medicine

The culture of medicine is such that individuals possessing certain character traits are actively recruited to the profession. Independence, hard work, stoicism, and selflessness are valued. Perfectionistic and compulsive characteristics are common in this population, as are a high need for achievement and an exaggerated sense of responsibility (Gabbard 1985). These characteristics are adaptive in medicine because clinicians need to be thorough and detail-oriented in order to minimize the risk of oversight and mistakes. Young people in medicine often have trouble saying no because they want to please everyone and have unrealistically high standards and expectations of themselves that are impossible to achieve and sustain across domains. Similar studies examining personality style and psychological adaptation in psychology trainees also suggest that there are significant numbers of individuals who have problems with anxiety and depression, which may be correlated with personality adjustment scores and may impact training and quality of life (Brooks et al. 2002). Another literature review concluded that psychology trainees are vulnerable to elevated stress. This stress, in turn, can negatively impact personal and professional functioning and may affect patient care (Pakenham and Stafford-Brown 2012).

Successful trainees in both psychiatry and psychology typically possess finely honed organization and executive function skills necessary to triage tasks appropriately, complete work efficiently, and balance competing interests between work and home life. When left unchecked, these qualities may lead to overwhelming feelings of isolation, crushing pressure, and excessive guilt. Trainees may feel as though they are not able to satisfy expectations at work and may also feel that they are letting family and friends down in their limited free time.

Risk of Mental Health Issues for Trainees

Students entering medical school have many strengths and, as a group, are no more likely than the general population to have exhibited mental health problems before training. A significant number of students develop symptoms of burnout or new psychiatric problems during training, and worsening mood is particularly common at defined points in the training process. Studies suggest that 20%–25% of medical students have been depressed (Rosenthal and Okie 2005), and 25%–35% of medical residents reported four to five symptoms of depression (Collier et al. 2002). Suicide is a growing problem (Lipkin 2019). Upward of 75% of residents in one study met criteria for burnout on the Maslach Burnout Inventory (Shanafelt et al. 2002). *Burnout*, described as the triad of emotional exhaustion, feelings of inadequacy, and depersonalization, can lead to compassion fatigue and poor patient outcomes and dissatisfaction (Beresin et al. 2016). Inadequately identified and treated mood and anxiety symptoms can lead to the development of other problematic health behaviors as clinicians attempt to self-manage symptoms through behaviors such as overeating or undereating, compulsive exercise, alcohol and/or drug use, gambling, or injudicious sexual behaviors.

Professional Stressors for Clinicians-in-Training

Many different aspects of the training environment can contribute to student stress. Medical errors, threats of litigation, examination failure, and secondary or vicarious traumatization due to hearing unsettling stories can have a particularly negative influence on student mental health (Coverdale et al. 2019). Caring for patients who are difficult, or even violent, as a trainee can lead to feelings of guilt and even loss of confidence (Coverdale et al. 2005), as illustrated in the following vignette.

Vignette

Janine Kerry-Smith, a new intern, was rotating on a behavioral neurology unit. She was on a multidisciplinary team that cared for patients with problems of aggression and impulsivity. Some of the patients had uncontrolled seizures, head injuries, and other neuropsychiatric disorders. One afternoon, a patient began screaming and gesturing angrily at Dr. Kerry-Smith. The crisis team was called, and the patient settled down, but the experience was upsetting to Dr. Kerry-Smith and other patients in the unit. The next morning, Dr. Kerry-Smith found herself dreading the idea of going to work. She became distressed while thinking of a night of on-call duties that would follow her daytime work on the unit. For the next several days, thoughts of the angry patient and the situation popped into her head, and she found herself feeling panicked when she approached the hospital each morning.

Difficult patients may be a stressful, but unavoidable, part of psychiatrists' and psychologists' careers even beyond training. Mental health care professionals who are verbally or physically assaulted by patients, families, or even other medical staff are at risk for posttraumatic stress disorder (Kannan et al. 2019). Despite increases in regulatory oversight, medical training is still rife with abuse from patients, staff, colleagues, and educators. Trainees continue to report public embarrassment, humiliation, gender discrimination, and unwanted sexual advances (Coverdale et al. 2009). Table 5–1 shows data from a systematic review and meta-analysis on the prevalence of harassment and discrimination for

TABLE 5–1. Prevalence of harassment and discrimination among physicians-in-training

	Number of studies and subjects	Prevalence	Type of trainees
Harassment	51 studies N=38,353	Mean 60% Range 11%–100%	More common for residents
Verbal abuse	28 studies N=27,258	Mean 63% Range 28%–94%	More common for students
Gender discrimination	13 studies N=6,237	Mean 54% Range 19%–92%	More common for residents
Sexual harassment	35 studies N=27,919	Mean 33% Range 3%–93%	Equally common for students and residents
Racial discrimination	10 studies N=19,455	Mean 24% Range 4%–58%	Equally common for students and residents
Physical abuse	24 studies N=23,776	Mean 15% Range 3%–100%	More common for residents

Source. Data from Fnais et al. 2014.

physicians-in-training (Fnais et al. 2014). Together, these issues highlight the seriousness of the types of stress trainees can face.

Training experiences that involve exposure to death or dying may force trainees to realize, for the first time, that continued medical treatment is sometimes futile despite best efforts. Experiencing the death of a patient for the first time can be a major source of stress. Although the death of a patient is difficult for any clinician, trainees and mental health professionals who experience the death of a patient from suicide face further challenges (House 2019). Trainees and mental health professionals who have lost a patient to suicide may struggle with guilt or self-blame and may lose confidence in their clinical skills, leading to avoidance of certain patient populations (Pilkinton and Etkin 2003).

In an effort to hear directly from trainees about their perceptions of factors like burnout and coping, Farquhar and colleagues conducted a focus group study of medical students in Singapore (Farquhar et al. 2018). The narratives provided by these students give powerful insight into their common experiences of stress and unique perspectives on resilience (see Table 5–2). These quotes make it clear that students are familiar with the concept of burnout and are actively grappling with the best ways of coping. Both professional issues encountered during training and personal issues related to the developmental stage of being a student challenge their mental health.

Personal Stressors for Clinicians-in-Training

Trainees are often, but not always, young. They come to training with varied life experiences. Some have extensive personal or community experience with injustice, trauma, or loss, whereas others are naive to adverse life events. Some trainees may be naturally optimistic and resilient. They may have had prior experiences that have made it necessary to develop adaptive coping strategies. Others may lack the basic coping strategies necessary to process even routine events in medical training. Physical and emotional health, a well-rounded education, and self-awareness of one's own background and personal characteristics help students thrive in training. Access to health care, intellectual resources, and a sense of community belonging are also critical for the positive growth of trainees. Figure 5–2 depicts some of the actions that help trainees become healers.

In addition to being new in their careers, medical trainees are often in the midst of significant developmental life milestones. Many individ-

TABLE 5–2. Student meaning of stress, burnout, coping, and resilience derived from focus group discussion

Meaning	Illustrative quote
Stress is a state of feeling pressured or uncomfortable and can involve physical symptoms. Stress can be negative or positive and can stem from external (time pressure, others' expectations) or internal (personal goals) sources.	"Stress is like a pressure or like a force." "Stress is when I feel uncomfortable when I'm faced with a situation." "Stress is decreased appetite and decreased sleep." "I think stress can be self-imposed or it can be put on you by others. I put a lot of stress on myself because of the expectations I have for myself." "There's a possibility that stress can be used in a good way."
Burnout is a sense of sustained physical and mental exhaustion, resulting in a depressed state, after pushing past one's limits.	"I think burnout is when you have been overwhelmed for a good amount of time." "You're exhausted, you lose your motivation…you don't care anymore." "Burnout is when you go beyond a certain threshold."
Coping is a manner of responding to and managing stress. Coping mechanisms are individual and can be active, passive, physical, and emotional.	"Coping is a method or way we deal with stress and stressful situations. I think people cope in different ways." "Some people are very clearly aware of their stress situation and they are actively doing something to relieve stress. But some others will just cope with the stress passively." "You can use [coping] in a physical or a psychological way."

TABLE 5–2. Student meaning of stress, burnout, coping, and resilience derived from focus group discussion (*continued*)

Meaning	Illustrative quote
Resilience is persisting in the face of stress or bouncing back from a negative experience. Resilience increases with experience and requires taking perspective and remembering one's goals.	"Resilience is the ability to make a comeback after a setback, like going beyond a failure." "Resilience to me is…how you face failure and what you can do to learn from the failure." "Think back to what makes you take on this decision in the first place…having that kind of goal…actually gives you resilience to move on further onto what you want to do."

Source. From Farquhar J, Lie D, Chan A, et al: Understanding medical students' experience with stress and its related constructs: a focus group study from Singapore. *Academic Psychiatry* 42(1):48–47, 2018. Reprinted with permission.

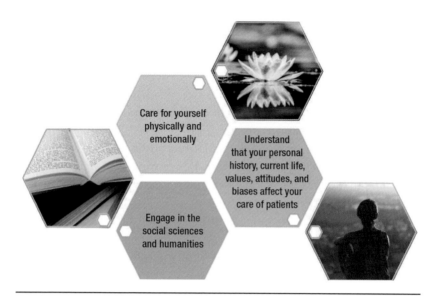

FIGURE 5–2. How to become a healer.

Source. Photo credits (left to right): Gabrielle Termuehlen, Michele Guan, and Christopher Sardegna.

uals move to new cities to attend school or start an internship, residency, or fellowship training and need to establish a new community or risk social isolation. Trainees may be coming to terms with sexual orientation and identity or preparing to come out, or they may be navigating new romantic relationships and cohabitating for the first time. They may need to manage personal or family illness or be faced with the stress of caring for ailing relatives. The busy years of medical training also often coincide with the "busyness" of life: marriage, childbearing, divorce, and child-rearing.

Medical education is also expensive, which can introduce tremendous stress into the lives of medical students, residents, and early-career physicians. A significant number of academic medical centers are located in cities with high costs of living, where it might be difficult to afford a comfortable lifestyle on a trainee salary. Trainees may need to moonlight in their free time in order to pay back large amounts of student debt. They may also realize that medicine was not actually the right career choice, after all, which could be devastating to someone facing a high-debt burden (Balch et al. 2009). The median 4-year cost of attending a public medical school in 2017 was $240,351, and the cost of a private medical school was $314,203 (Marcu et al. 2017). Most medical students entering residency reported significant educational debt in 2018. The median amount of combined college and medical school debt, for those individuals with debt, was $200,000. Many students may still be years away from making a comfortable salary, with debt appearing to shape decisions regarding the type of practice that residents choose to pursue. Residents with higher debt are less likely, for example, to enter academia or to work for a government organization.

Even with 80-hour workweek regulations put in place by the Accreditation Council for Graduate Medical Education (ACGME), workdays are long, call days are busy, and there may not be adequate time outside training to cultivate meaningful work or activities that bring joy. Sleep, exercise, and proper nutrition may suffer because of long hours spent in the hospital and/or clinic.

With regard to leave time, there is significant inequality between faculty and resident physicians. A recent study of 12 top U.S. medical schools demonstrated that the mean paid childbearing leave for faculty physicians was 8.6 weeks, compared with a mean duration of 6.6 weeks paid maternity leave for residents at the same institutions (Magudia et al. 2018). Only about half of the ACGME-sponsored programs had policies providing paid leave for trainees, although all had such policies for faculty. The American Academy of Pediatrics supports a proposed federal law providing 12 paid weeks (Magudia et al. 2018).

Trainees and Preexisting Mental Health Challenges

With improved identification and treatment of psychiatric illness early in life, increasing numbers of trainees may arrive at training programs with previous mental health diagnoses already in place. Trainees with a history of mental health issues may struggle with the decision to enter the mental health field and may feel conflicted about deciding whether to disclose their experiences to training programs. Although many prospective trainees may feel that their own experiences have shaped their decision to pursue a particular career path and will help them become more empathic and sensitive clinicians, they might worry about the implications of openly discussing their motivations (Brenner et al. 2018). They may also be concerned about their ability to complete training or worry that they are reinforcing the cliché that people who pursue a career in the mental health professions are solely seeking to cure themselves. For example, 21% of fourth-year medical students who were interviewed expressed belief that individuals going into psychiatry were "broken in the head" (Cutler et al. 2009). Psychiatrists and psychologists who need to take medical leave may grapple with how to explain gaps in education or extended time to complete the curriculum.

The demands of training and perceived time pressure make it tempting for learners to discontinue psychiatric care, attempt to self-prescribe, or rely on "curbside consultations" from colleagues rather than accessing their own treatments. Some trainees may find it difficult to devote the time necessary for appointments, whereas others may hope that this new phase of life will afford an opportunity for a "fresh start," free from the need for mental health treatment. Asking for help or time off can be worrisome, especially when struggling with stigma and fears that medical competence or devotion to the field will be questioned (Roberts 2009).

Program administration may also be conflicted about accepting a trainee with a history of mental health difficulties into their program. Most individuals would agree that experiencing any sort of illness does not preclude a career in medicine. The experience of being a patient can bring rich benefit to one's clinical work. At the same time, predicting whether someone will experience a relapse during training is difficult. Although the Americans with Disabilities Act prevents training programs from asking about personal health history that was not initially brought up by the trainee, program directors may be concerned that an applicant with a mental health history may have trouble completing the program. The stress of training, including sleep deprivation while on call, may put trainees at risk of relapse. Programs (and applicants themselves) worry about stressing colleagues who might be called on to take over call responsibilities or to provide coverage at critical clinical sites. Program directors may also worry about gaps in learning and memory during times of increased symptoms and professionalism issues, such as injudicious self-disclosure and other boundary crossings that may put patients at risk (Brenner et al. 2018).

Solutions for the Future

Reframing the culture of medicine may be the only way to change trainees' unrealistic expectations of themselves. It is neither helpful nor acceptable for senior physicians to insist that learners continue to be trained in the same toxic culture simply because "we did it and it made us stronger." Through didactic lectures and small-group discussions allowing for individual reflection, there needs to be explicit acknowledgment that the temperamental traits valued in medical training are also very real risk factors for burnout and may develop into more serious mental health conditions. Clinicians need to be acutely aware of the challenges trainees face and actively work to ensure that they are adequately supported. New trainees may benefit from communications early on (even right after they match with a new clinical placement), by encouraging continuation with treatment for any chronic medical or mental health conditions. Supplying trainees with a list of local health professionals would also be encouraging and beneficial. Easy access to appointments and protected time away from rotations is important for trainees to feel comfortable taking time for self-care (Table 5–3).

Programs can provide trainees with opportunities to develop more effective and adaptive coping and time management strategies as part of the required curriculum in professionalism. Mental health professionals should explicitly point out and correct the black-and-white thinking that may pervade medical training (Table 5–4). For example, instead of saying, "I have to do everything, and it must be perfect," it is more realistic and healthier to say, "I need to do my best to cover all of the important things on my list, and I can ask other members of my team for help." Instead of an "eat when you can, sleep when you must" attitude, mental health professionals should shift the focus to "adequate rest and nutrition are important to have enough mental and physical energy to do my job well. My patients depend on me to take good care of myself."

Resilience can be taught and developed with the appropriate scaffolding in place. Offering experiences for trainees to practice dealing with stresses from early on in medical school, rather than "protecting" the most inexperienced trainees from adverse outcomes or traumatic experiences, may be valuable. Allowing trainees to participate in, process, and take meaning from adverse situations with other members of the team provides an enriching experience instead of the inadvertent message that they are too fragile to handle sensitive and difficult topics.

When trainees experience the onset or relapse of mental health symptoms, their training program should respond appropriately. Focus should be placed on behaviors and professionalism issues rather than diagnoses, and the faculty should resist the urge to be pulled into clinical treatment if at all possible. Working with the institution's graduate medical education office may be necessary to negotiate the terms of a medical leave or to assist in formulating a remediation plan. The program should have a safety net in place (e.g., a jeopardy on-call system) to cover the duties of the affected trainee, and the individual's colleagues should be allowed the opportunity to process their feelings and experiences in a safe

TABLE 5–3.	Suggested communication to trainees prior to starting program

Right after students match with a new training program, send email normalizing the stress of training and encouraging trainees to seek out (or continue) appropriate mental health support.

Provide a list of local primary care doctors, psychiatrists, and therapists to encourage early connection to care.

Encourage the development of hobbies and activities outside training to promote relaxation and adaptive coping.

Discuss the importance of cultivating and nurturing important relationships throughout the training process.

Provide explicit wellness resources available on campus for students, interns, residents, and fellows.

TABLE 5–4. Reframing unhelpful thinking

Unhelpful thinking	Helpful thinking
"I must get everything done myself."	"I need to prioritize the most important things. I can ask for help with the others."
"I do not have time to sleep or take any breaks."	"I will be better able to care for my patients if I am well rested."
"There is no time to buy fresh groceries or prepare a meal from scratch."	"Taking the time to prepare and enjoy a homemade meal is good modeling of healthy behaviors."
"If my patient does not do well, I am a failure."	"Sometimes, despite our best efforts, people do not recover."
"If I make a mistake, I am an awful person."	"I am human, and sometimes humans make errors."

forum (Brenner et al. 2018). The following case examples further illustrate how personal and professional challenges during training can place student well-being in jeopardy and how a diverse set of supports is needed to maximize positive outcomes for students, the mental health community, and the general public.

Case Example 1

Leslie Harris is a third-year medical student (about halfway through the year) in a rigorous medical school located across the country from her home. She attended an undergraduate institution near her parents so that she could care for her elderly grandparents, who have since passed away. She has always been an excellent student, with top grades in her class, and has stood out in all of her extracurricular activities. With the transition to medical school, she has found herself in an unfamiliar situation. Although her classmates are friendly, a majority have developed relationships with others in class because most of them completed undergraduate work at the same university where the medical school is located. Many students also share a similar socioeconomic and family background, which is different from hers. Leslie is a first-generation college student, supported by loans and scholarships and the love of her proud parents. She has not had the experience of summer camps and prestigious boarding schools that many of her classmates have had. Her grades are average for her class, but she has never before had the experience of not being a "star."

Leslie came to medical school with dreams of specializing in geriatric psychiatry. She found it troubling that there were so few clinicians who felt comfortable caring for her grandparents once they started to show evidence of cognitive decline. She is the only member of her class who is openly interested in pursuing psychiatry, and she finds that classmates and faculty are somewhat dismissive of her career plans. On her surgery rotation, an attending she was assisting said, "Oh, you're too smart for that, you'll see the light," when he heard that Leslie was planning a psychiatry residency. While a psychiatry attending was giving a lecture on the assessment and treatment of psychosis, a group of classmates snickered with a peer who whispered, "They're only willing to work with those people because they have 'issues' too."

Leslie is unhappy and worried that she made a mistake when she applied to medical school. She notes worsening low mood, anhedonia, fatigue, and social isolation. She does not feel like going out but follows a number of classmates on social media and is disappointed when she sees posts documenting parties and gatherings she was not invited to join. She has never contemplated suicide. She is just not sure whether she should see the training through or if she should just "cut losses and go home."

Leslie's mother encourages her to meet with her academic advisor to review her options. They discuss the possibility of Leslie transferring to a medical school closer to home, as well as the pros and cons of completing the program versus quitting outright. They also arrange for her to meet with a local geriatric psychiatrist, who is willing to share her experiences of training and was honest about the practicalities and realities of her career. The psychiatrist invites Leslie to shadow her while she makes rounds at a local inpatient dementia unit.

Leslie ultimately decides to stay in medical school but transfers to a program near home, where she feels more comfortable and is able to reconnect with her friends. She decides that, at the very least, if she ends up not liking residency and fellowship, she can find ways to make her degree work in a nonclinical role.

This case of Leslie Harris highlights a number of common issues for medical students. Leslie has always worked hard and has excelled in return, but she finds that the stakes are much higher in medical school, and she must come to terms with being "average," even though she is working hard. In addition, she is far from home and is having trouble connecting with other students whose background and interests differ from hers. Students have a wide range of ethnic, cultural, and socioeconomic histories. Individuals who move from other areas of the country likely experience additional stresses acclimating to the increased academic rigor while transitioning from undergraduate education to medical school. Further compounding the situation, Leslie experiences negativity about her chosen specialty, which causes her to question her career path. She finds it helpful to connect with an advisor to realistically consider her options and to seek career mentors to better understand her future.

Case Example 2

John Chamberlin is a second-year general psychiatry resident. Dr. Chamberlin made a comment in process group, stating, "Residency sucks. I'm not sleeping. I'm eating crap. I drink too much, and I find it kind of hilarious that I'm trying to help people with almost exactly the same issues." Several members of the group reacted with concern, and the leader referred Dr. Chamberlin for assessment. Dr. Chamberlin was angry with the group leader and his peers for sharing their concerns because he had felt safe enough within the group to share his true feelings. He felt dismayed that his confidentiality and privacy had been betrayed.

Dr. Chamberlin attended an assessment session but was fairly terse in his answers. Although he was offered ongoing therapy sessions, he declined. He continued to show up for work on the inpatient unit each day, but there was concern about his work performance. He frequently showed up late, fell asleep during rounds, or disappeared for long periods of time during the day. He could be difficult to reach when there were questions on the unit. One night, his co-resident was called after hours to help out with a question on the unit because Dr. Chamberlin was not responding to pages even though he had been identified as being on call that evening.

One day, his attending decided to send him home for the day after he fell asleep during rounds and blamed it on new medication he was taking. The attending was clear that Dr. Chamberlin needed the rest, was not in an appropriate state to care for patients, and should see this as an opportunity to practice good self-care. The attending also notified the program director, who mentioned that there had been other concerns raised by an outpatient supervisor that made her think more needed to be done to address the issue. Higher-level administration within the institution's graduate medical education office was notified, conducted a thorough review of the situation, and recommended that Dr. Chamberlin take a medical leave to focus on suspected mood and substance issues, with very clear expectations that would need to be met in order for him to return to the training program. Dr. Chamberlin was furious and threatened legal action against the program. He followed the recommendation that he take medical leave, completed treatment, and ultimately decided not to return to the training program. Instead, he joined a medical consulting firm.

Dr. Chamberlin's situation is concerning. Red flags in his work performance indicate possible impairment and warrant additional information. His supervisors and peers are in the difficult position of reporting concerning behavior despite the fact that Dr. Chamberlin is resistant to help and hostile to colleagues who express concern for him. In situations like these, it is important to consult with the institution's graduate medical education office to ensure that the appropriate steps are taken to protect patient care, while also making sure to document the steps taken to offer remediation and assistance. Mental health professionals should demonstrate that any actions taken are not retaliatory in nature and that there is no evidence of discrimination based on an underlying mental health diagnosis. It is entirely possible for a motivated trainee to complete a recommended treatment program, participate in ongoing monitoring, and return to training with appropriate scaffolding and support in place. Other individuals may decide that the ability to complete training and practice medicine is not worth the added stress. Still, trainees may find that, despite motivation, the degree of illness precludes completion of training.

Positive Practices

1. Recognize that medical students and residents are uniquely vulnerable. Not only are they at the age when many severe mental illnesses first declare themselves, but they are immersed in an incredibly high stress environment, which can increase the likelihood that symptoms will develop in those who are genetically predisposed.
2. As supervisors and clinicians working with medical students, residents, and fellows, be aware that many times these young people are in the midst of big life transitions in addition to managing the stresses of a busy clinical practice. They are often caring for the sickest patients while also dealing with their own developmental growing pains.

These issues include recent geographic relocation, attempts to build a social life in their new city, romantic relationships, marriage, and decisions about childbearing and child-rearing.

3. Acknowledge that medical students and physicians-in-training may have even more difficulty than attending physicians with asking for help and prioritizing health and wellness. They are often hesitant to burden their attending physicians or other members of their team and are working hard to earn the glowing evaluations that will be necessary to earn a coveted residency, fellowship, or faculty position.

4. Although the governing bodies responsible for regulating graduate medical education have made progress in shifting the culture of medicine, remnants of the older culture remain. Independence, stoicism, and the ability to withstand intense situations without extraneous emotion have long been qualities celebrated in young doctors. Continue to encourage trainees and early-career physicians to be reflective and willing to debrief their experiences and rely on their community for support.

Conclusion

Trainees in health care—particularly medical students, residents, psychology graduate students, interns, and postdoctoral fellows—are vulnerable to anxiety, depression, substance use, and other mental health issues that can negatively impact their personal and professional lives. Individuals attracted to the helping professions tend to be passionate and caring and also perfectionistic and achievement focused. Age, temperament, developmental stage, and previous life experiences influence resiliency and the ability to adjust to the difficulties inherent in training in a high-stress environment. Efforts to shift the culture of medicine to encourage adequate self-care and promote the development of resiliency may protect the longevity of clinician careers and lead to improved patient outcomes.

Questions to Discuss With Colleagues and Mentors
———————o———————

- What can we do in everyday interactions to nurture trainee health and well-being?
- How can I model good self-care practices with students, residents, interns, and fellows?
- What stresses are trainees in the system most concerned about?

- What supports and threats exist in the training environment that can affect trainee well-being?
- What supports during training were most helpful to my professional well-being, and how can I put these supports into practice for current trainees?

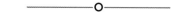

Recommended Resources

Accreditation Council for Graduate Medical Education: ACGME tools and resources for resident and faculty member well-being. Chicago, IL, Accreditation Council for Graduate Medical Education, 2018. Available at: www.acgme.org/What-We-Do/Initiatives/Physician-Well-Being/Resources. Accessed December 12, 2019.

American Medical Student Association: Medical student well-being. Chantilly, VA, American Medical Student Association, 2019. Available at: www.amsa.org/advocacy/action-committees/twp/well-being. Accessed December 12, 2019.

Association of American Medical Colleges: Well-being in academic medicine: resources for faculty. Washington, DC, Association of American Medical Colleges, 2019. Available at: www.aamc.org/initiatives/462280/well-being-academic-medicine.html. Accessed December 12, 2019.

Konner M: Becoming a Doctor: A Journey of Initiation in Medical School. New York, Penguin, 1988

Marion R: The Intern Blues: The Private Ordeals of Three Young Doctors. New York, Morrow, 1989

Peterkin AD: Staying Human During Residency Training: How to Survive and Thrive After Medical School. Toronto, ON, Canada, University of Toronto Press, 2016

Roberts LW: Understanding depression and distress among medical students. JAMA 304(11):1231–1233, 2010

Virshup B: Coping in Medical School. Chapel Hill, NC, Health Sciences Consortium, 1981

References

Balch CM, Freischlag JA, Shanafelt TD: Stress and burnout among surgeons: understanding and managing the syndrome and avoiding the adverse consequences. Arch Surg 144(4):371–376, 2009 19380652

Beresin EV, Milligan TA, Balon R, et al: Physician wellbeing: a critical deficiency in resilience education and training. Acad Psychiatry 40(1):9–12, 2016 26691141

Brenner AM, Balon R, Guerrero AP, et al: Training as a psychiatrist when having a psychiatric illness, Acad Psychiatry 42(5):592–597, 2018

Brooks J, Holttum S, Lavender A: Personality style, psychological adaptation and expectations of trainee clinical psychologists. Clinical Psychol Psychotherapy 9(4):253–270, 2002

Collier V, McCue J, Markus A, et al: Stress in medical residency: status quo after a decade of reform? Ann Intern Med 136(5):384–390, 2002 11874311

Coverdale JH, Louie AK, Roberts LW: Protecting the safety of medical students and residents. Acad Psychiatry 29(4):329–331, 2005 16223893

Coverdale JH, Balon R, Roberts LW: Mistreatment of trainees: verbal abuse and other bullying behaviors. Acad Psychiatry 33(4):269–273, 2009 19690101

Coverdale J, Balon R, Beresin EV, et al: What are some stressful adversities in psychiatry residency training, and how should they be managed professionally?Acad Psychiatry 43(2):145–150, 2019 30697662

Cutler JL, Harding KJ, Mozian SA, et al: Discrediting the notion "working with 'crazies' will make you 'crazy'": addressing stigma and enhancing empathy in medical student education. Adv Health Sci Educ Theory Pract 14(4):487–502, 2009 18766453

Farquhar J, Lie D, Chan A, et al: Understanding medical students' experience with stress and its related constructs: a focus group study from Singapore. Acad Psychiatry 42(1):48–57, 2018 28421479

Fnais N, Soobiah C, Chen MH, et al: Harassment and discrimination in medical training: a systematic review and meta-analysis. Acad Med 89(5):817–827, 2014 24667512

Gabbard GO: The role of compulsiveness in the normal physician. JAMA 254(20):2926–2929, 1985 4057513

House A: Suicide and the psychiatrist: commentary on... effects of patient suicide on psychiatrists. BJPsych Bulletin 43(5):242–244, 2019

Huprich SK, Rudd MD: A national survey of trainee impairment in clinical, counseling, and school psychology doctoral programs and internships. J Clin Psychol 60(1):43–52, 2004 14692008

Kannan L, Wheeler DS, Blumhof S, et al: Work related post traumatic stress disorder in medicine residents. Acad Psychiatry 43(2):167–170, 2019 29644602

Lipkin M: When suicide happens in the medical community. J Gen Intern Med 34(2):317–319, 2019 30426344

Magudia K, Bick A, Cohen J, et al: Childbearing and family leave policies for resident physicians at top training institutions. JAMA 320(22):2372–2374, 2018 30535210

Marcu MI, Kellermann AL, Hunter C, et al: Borrow or serve? An economic analysis of options for financing a medical school education. Acad Med 92(7):966–975, 2017 28121649

Pakenham KI, Stafford-Brown J: Stress in clinical psychology trainees: current research status and future directions. Australian Psychologist 47(3):147–155, 2012

Pilkinton P, Etkin M: Encountering suicide: the experience of psychiatric residents. Acad Psychiatry 27(2):93–99, 2003 12824109

Roberts LW: Hard duty. Acad Psychiatry 33(4):274–277, 2009 19690103

Roberts LW: Understanding depression and distress among medical students. JAMA 304(11):1231–1233, 2010 20841539

Rosenthal JM, Okie S: White coat, mood indigo—depression in medical school. N Engl J Med 353(11):1085–1088, 2005 16162877

Salsberg E, Grover A: Physician workforce shortages: implications and issues for academic health centers and policymakers. Acad Med 81(9):782–787, 2006 16936479

Shanafelt TD, Bradley KA, Wipf JE, Back AL: Burnout and self-reported patient care in an internal medicine residency program. Ann Intern Med 136(5):358–367, 2002 11874308

CHAPTER 6

Systems and Supports for Clinician Wellness

The issue of healthy work environments is appropriately receiving increased attention across major organizations. For instance, the American Psychological Association Center for Organizational Excellence is now offering awards for psychologically healthy workplaces and for organizational excellence to honor employers who have implemented workplace practices designed to foster employee well-being and enhance organizational performance. The unique challenges in providing mental health care are also increasingly acknowledged (Rupert et al. 2015), prompting large health care organizations to turn attention to supporting the well-being of psychiatrists, psychologists, and other mental health clinicians. These developments have positive effects for mental health professionals because systems that adequately support clinicians are more likely to have high levels of clinician engagement and professional fulfillment (Schaufeli et al. 2009; Wise et al. 2012).

Although some systems support individual well-being, other systems offer support at the organizational level and impact clinicians across disciplines (Awa et al. 2010; Panagioti et al. 2017; Regehr et al. 2014). Actions can be taken by individual practitioners and by organizational leaders to support the well-being of mental health professionals (LoboPrabhu et al. 2020; West et al. 2015). In this chapter, we focus on the ways that problems with clinician wellness can be viewed as a system-wide issue, the business case for intervening to enhance professional engagement, and common practices to support wellness in the workplace and program models integrating intervention and prevention efforts.

The Problem of Professional Wellness as a Systems Issue

Health care systems need clinicians to be engaged, resilient, and committed to improving quality and efficiency of care (Shanafelt and Noseworthy 2017). Although burnout and compromised well-being take a serious toll on individual clinicians, these symptoms also have widespread implications across the health care system (Harris et al. 2006; Santos et al. 2010; Weinberg and Creed 2000). Stress can impact a clinician's concentration, decision-making, communication skills, and capacity for empathy, all of which are critical for effective patient care (Beddoe and Murphy 2004; Enochs and Etzbach 2004; Irving et al. 2009; Skosnik et al. 2000). As discussed in detail in the preceding chapters, professional burnout in medical contexts has been repeatedly shown to be related to patient safety, care quality, and patient satisfaction (Cimiotti et al. 2012; de Oliveira et al. 2013; Firth-Cozens and Greenhalgh 1997; Haas et al. 2000; Shanafelt and Noseworthy 2017; Shanafelt et al. 2002, 2010; Tawfik et al. 2017; Welp et al. 2015; West et al. 2006, 2009; Williams et al. 2007). For instance, poor self-care among health care professionals heightens the risk of medical errors (Hall et al. 2016). Burnout also influences professional work effort and turnover (Dewa et al. 2014; Shanafelt et al. 2011b; Williams et al. 2002, 2010). Key drivers of physician well-being are manageable workload and job demands, control and flexibility, efficiency and resources, work-life integration, organizational culture and values, meaning in work, and social support and sense of community at work (Konrad et al. 1999; Shanafelt 2009; Shanafelt and Noseworthy 2017; Shanafelt et al. 2016b; Wallace et al. 2009). When these factors are problematic, burnout can result. When they are optimal, engagement is more likely.

In clinical training contexts, faculty wellness impacts the training experiences of students under their supervision. For example, medical school faculty who experience burnout may place more pressure on the residents, who, in turn, may be less supportive with the medical students they supervise (Irving et al. 2009). The following vignette illustrates how problematic resident stress can be for students they supervise.

Vignette

Nisha Kahn was excited to start her first clinical rotation as a medical student. When she learned that she would be working in the hospital's pediatric inpatient psychiatry program, she was nervous about meeting children who had been hospitalized for such severe behavior, but she also was curious because she had always wondered if she might like to become a child psychiatrist. On her first day, she was assigned to shadow Dr. John Pence, one of the child psychiatry fellows working on the unit. The first time they met, she was impressed by how much Dr. Pence seemed to know about the patients' symptoms, treatments, and discharge options. Unfortunately, he did not seem to have time to explain or teach much of this information to her. The more she watched him, the more she could see how much pressure he was under from the unit's attending psychiatrist to admit new patients quickly and make sure each patient on his large caseload was making progress toward discharge. She remembered that there had been a recent newspaper article about the inpatient unit, which criticized the program for being poorly run and always too full to take children in crisis. She could tell that this bad press was making everyone feel frazzled and misunderstood. Wanting to help and learn, she worked side by side with Dr. Pence day after day, drafting notes, making phone calls, meeting with the patients, and attending daily rounds. Still, he never seemed to have the patience to answer questions when she did not know how to do something. He would usually say something about how "no one ever gave me any handouts when I was in med school" and "maybe if they gave me a few days off, I could catch up on all this work." One time during rounds, when she made a mistake in describing the patient's updated treatment plan, he lost his temper and yelled, "Dammit, I guess I just have to do everything myself around here!" and stormed out of the room. She was devastated and started thinking that maybe she should not pursue psychiatry after all.

Professional well-being is not the sole responsibility of the individual health care professional (Demerouti et al. 2001; Scheurer et al. 2009). When physicians are directed to pursue interventions individually, they may feel blamed or blame themselves for being less resilient (Panagioti et al. 2017; Swensen et al. 2016). Wellness programming can even exacerbate discrimination against professionals who may already be struggling at work (Kirkland 2014). Solutions focused on improving the resilience of individual clinicians can fail to address the core drivers of burnout and may be viewed with skepticism by professionals they are designed to help (Shanafelt and Noseworthy 2017). Although targeted interventions have been shown to yield important benefits, they may not be sufficient to produce widespread changes in workforce functioning (Baker and Sen 2016). As shown in Table 6–1, workplace distress can have negative consequences both for the individual and throughout the work group. System-level interventions are also necessary to support and sustain an engaged professional workforce (Panagioti et al. 2017).

TABLE 6–1. Negative consequences of workplace distress and sources of professional burnout

Individual	Work group
Personal anguish, anxiety, exhaustion	Low morale
Potential for poor performance	Lowered productivity
Potential for decreased productivity	Colleague disengagement
Taking more time off	Staff turnover
Working despite stress or illness	Overwork to compensate for burned-out colleagues
Lessened opportunities as a positive role model	
Job insecurity	Negative workplace-related attitudes affecting new hires

A recent meta-analysis of interventions for physicians concluded that organizational interventions were as effective, and in some cases more effective, than individual interventions for reducing overall burnout (West et al. 2016). Adjusting workload and schedule, involving clinicians in decision-making, and providing mentorship can all help protect against burnout (Panagioti et al. 2017). The provision of mental health care places particular kinds of stress on clinicians (Lee et al. 2011; Lim et al. 2010). The urgent needs of patients in emotional crisis are compelling and sometimes frightening, which places strong pressure on clinicians to work above and beyond their normal limitations. Viewing professional wellness as a system-wide problem gives appropriate responsibility to multiple sources of strain and makes it clear that effective interventions must be developed with the relevant contextual influences in mind.

A growing body of evidence suggests that clinician burnout in health care systems is related to many organizational factors (LoboPrabhu et al. 2020; Panagioti et al. 2017; Sharp and Stevens 2019; West and Hauer 2015). One potent example is that near-universal adoption of electronic health records (EHRs) in large medical systems has changed the day-to-day experience of providing health care and may further burden clinicians and exacerbate the problems of burnout (DiAngi et al. 2017). Although in many industries the increased use of technology has improved work efficiency, practitioners using EHRs often experience more clerical burden (Shanafelt et al. 2016a; Sinsky et al. 2016).

Skilled leadership is critical for the resilience of mental health professionals. By providing clarity of vision and direction to group effort, leaders can energize and empower their staff to work productively toward a common goal and achieve meaningful impact. Leadership skill has been shown to influence both burnout and satisfaction. For instance, in a study of more than 2,800 physicians at the Mayo Clinic, 11% of the variance in burnout between work units and 47% of the variance in satisfaction was attributable to the leadership ratings supervisors received from their physician staff (Shanafelt et al. 2015a). In recognition of the important role of leadership in enhancing physician well-being, the National Academy of Medicine has created a Clinician Well-Being Knowledge Hub (https://nam.edu/clinicianwellbeing), providing public acknowledgment that progress depends on involvement of executive leadership and staff at all levels with open exchange of information.

Measuring professional burnout and engagement across the organization and at regular intervals is also helpful for understanding the scope of the problem, developing solutions, and monitoring impact. If burnout is found to be significant, open acknowledgment of this fact by leadership is critical, as well as having the commitment to engage in targeted interventions. Staff at all levels within the organization should be included in discussions and planning efforts. The following vignette provides an example of an organization that identified elevated rates of clinician burnout and implemented leadership interventions to begin addressing the problem.

Vignette

Jill Sanchez has been clinical director of an outpatient mental health clinic for 3 years. The clinic services have been expanding rapidly, and she has recently hired several new psychologists, social workers, and a psychiatrist. The opportunity Dr. Sanchez likes most about her role is being able to mentor new clinicians as they begin their careers. The clinic is embedded within a large primary care health network, which serves a mix of patients from the nearby city as well as surrounding rural areas. The network has recently kicked off a clinician wellness campaign, starting with a company-wide survey of all staff to assess burnout and professional engagement. When Dr. Sanchez receives the results of the survey, she learns that, although the agency as a whole has a significant problem of clinician burnout, the staff in her mental health clinic are reporting even higher levels of distress than the agency mean. Her boss offers to meet with her to discuss the results and brainstorm possible interventions. During this meeting, Dr. Sanchez raises the concern that the pressures of the job seem to be particularly difficult for women on her team. The survey data also indicate that staff from racial and ethnic minority groups are disproportionately burned out. In the meeting, Dr. Sanchez and her supervisor identify several next steps to consider:

1. Making confidential counselors available to clinicians with high levels of burnout
2. Initiating a feasibility analysis to determine whether opening the clinic for weekend and evening sessions is financially viable, which would allow employees more flexible scheduling options for meeting clinical care targets
3. Convening a diverse group of employees to provide feedback on how the clinic can better support minority staff
4. Weekly leadership coaching sessions for Dr. Sanchez to learn about how she can adjust her leadership style to better support employees she supervises and encourage their professional engagement

Individuals from racial, ethnic, sexual, and gender minority groups may be underrepresented in many professional positions and may experience additional institutional barriers to professional success and even greater risk of burnout. National surveys have indicated that women physicians may report rates of burnout 60% higher than for men (Shanafelt et al. 2012b, 2016a). Clinicians from underrepresented minorities may also be at increased risk of burnout. These factors highlight how the need to address professional burnout is even more urgent given its disproportionate effect on those who are already vulnerable (Linzer et al. 2014).

Special Challenges in Low-Resource Settings

Clinicians working in systems with few resources can also be at elevated risk for burnout. Often, small clinics or clinics operating in rural or inner-city areas may have too few staff, tightly constrained finances, and limited ability to make changes in support of clinician wellness. In addition, demand for clinician time is often quite intense in these settings, and clinical acuity can be high when patients have minimal access to other health care professionals or types of support. When a clinician is confronted on a daily basis with the reality that there is no way to meet the needs of all the patients who require care, the feeling can be demoralizing. Unfortunately, the high rates of burnout in these settings drive higher clinician turnover, exacerbating troubling discrepancies in quality and continuity of care for racial or ethnic minority patients and other historically underserved populations.

The burden of trying to address such a wide variety of patient needs (e.g., transportation, housing, food, clothes, employment, legal aid) in addition to necessary mental health care can be immense. For this reason, clinicians practicing in low-resource settings, as well as administrators and policy makers who aim to support them, must be creative in seeking solutions relevant to their practice setting. Innovative programs can be born of necessity, and many new models of care have emerged that are successful with limited funding, precisely because they were created in spite of the lack of systemic resources. As outlined in the following vignette, when there is no way to meet the full need in a community, working together to figure out how to do the most good with what resources are available can be a powerful intervention. In spite of seemingly infinite need, it is comforting to know that the work can be meaningful and collaboration opportunities are possible with a team of people who care deeply.

Vignette

Gary Burz serves as a child and adolescent psychiatry fellow working on call in the only 24/7/365 psychiatric emergency department in a rural state. The local community was hit hard by unemployment, poverty, and immigration issues. Every night Dr. Burz was on duty, he felt more overwhelmed with the distress of the families he met who were seeking crisis services. The nurses, residents, and consulting physicians worked hard and genuinely cared about the patients, but everyone seemed to feel discouraged by the number of patients in need and the lack of mental health services available in their community. It seemed as if no matter how hard they worked, there was no way to make enough of a difference for the families who were suffering so much.

When a new psychologist, Dr. Sandra Judson, moved to the area and started meeting her colleagues, she could see how demoralized the health care professionals were feeling. She proposed a new model of care and suggested the development of a multidisciplinary clinic to provide short-term care for families in need of mental health services. The idea was to provide walk-in, clinic-based crisis intervention, which would keep families from having to access mental health care through emergency department visits. Dr. Judson advocated for clinicians in the new clinic to focus on three critical goals: 1) help families build on their strengths in order to cope with the stresses they were facing; 2) avoid sending suicidal adolescents to neighboring states for expensive, "revolving door" psychiatric hospitalizations; and 3) emphasize culturally attuned care by involving critical family members in intervention whenever possible.

With greater clarity of purpose and a team approach, the clinicians began to feel that they were making a difference with what few resources they had. Dr. Burz and his colleagues in the emergency department and the crisis clinic felt excitement about the new model of care for distressed families in the area and a renewed sense of optimism through working together for this common purpose.

A feeling of belonging among staff, whether through mentorship or peer support, is especially critical when other resources are not available. Clinicians operating in low-resource settings may be advised to make special efforts to form alliances with colleagues around a common purpose. Many times, the most successful programs succeed not because of unlimited resources but because of people working closely together, pursuing clear and strategic goals, giving what they have, and doing their best. When doing hard work, the feeling of not being alone can make a difference for morale and sense of fulfillment.

The Business Case for Clinician Well-Being

Successful health systems must focus on 1) providing high-quality care and 2) improving patient outcomes while 3) keeping costs in check. Consequently, many systems are pivoting to simultaneously focus on a fourth goal, clinician wellness, given the impact on quality of care, patient satisfaction, and cost (Bodenheimer and Sinsky 2014). Practicing clinicians in an agency can be considered the organization's most valuable asset in pursuing its mission. Although estimating the financial impact of healthy workplaces can be difficult, data are now emerging supporting the business case for investment in clinician wellness (MacKinnon and Murray 2018; Shanafelt and Noseworthy 2017).

Outside the health care field, there is growing acknowledgment that a climate of psychosocial safety has business benefits. For instance, a 2016 Safe Work Australia government report showed that workers in environments with high levels of psychological safety had managers who took emotional health of employees into account and designed roles to include reasonable demands, as well as autonomy and social support (Becher and Dollard 2016). In contrast, workers in environments with high demands and low control were 43% more likely to take sick days or show low productivity on the job. In addition, there is growing appreciation of the fact that specific workplace policies can enhance retention and productivity. A longitudinal study of workers in the United Kingdom indicated that although many of the women surveyed had reduced their working hours after a child was born, women who set their own working hours were significantly less likely to reduce their work commitments when returning to work after maternity leave (Chung and van der Horst 2018).

As in any business, the practical realities of providing mental health care are constantly changing. Health care systems must evolve to accommodate new standards of care, evidence-based practices, health care legislation, insurance policies, and new technologies (Shanafelt and Noseworthy 2017). Aspects of these changes can enhance clinician well-being but also can bring additional strain to an already fragile workforce. In the context of a rapidly changing knowledge base and increasing regulatory require-ments, reduced professional autonomy and greater expectations regarding workload and productivity are serious risk factors (Shanafelt et al. 2017). For physicians and mental health professionals who bill for patient care activities, compensation models have a major effect on risk of burnout. Productivity-based compensation can have a particular effect on physi-cian burnout because clinicians may feel pressure to work longer hours rather than compromising quality of care to improve efficiency or revenue generation (Shanafelt and Noseworthy 2017).

Burnout and turnover also have direct financial costs for health care systems (Dewa et al. 2014; Shanafelt et al. 2011b, 2014). When a clinician experiences burnout and leaves the work environment, that employee must typically be replaced. A recent case study of physicians within Stan-ford's hospitals indicated that physicians experiencing burnout had a 168% greater chance of leaving their jobs within 2 years than did those who were not experiencing burnout (Hamidi et al. 2018). Replacing clini-cians is often difficult and can be expensive (Alameddine et al. 2009). Estimates have indicated that when recruitment, onboarding, and lost revenue are considered, the actual costs of replacing a physician may be two to three times the physician's annual salary (Shanafelt and Nosewor-thy 2017). During this time, patient access to care is compromised. Re-cent estimates indicate that physician turnover and reduced clinical hours alone may cost U.S. health care organizations as much as $4.6 billion an-nually, which is about $7,600 per employed physician (Han et al. 2019).

Even if clinicians remain employed, excessive sick leave costs the or-ganization. Employed workers who show reduced productivity due to burnout place a further financial strain on the system. Lower levels of employee engagement and commitment are also difficult to quantify, but they certainly reduce a system's profitability. A study of 2,000 physi-cians at the Mayo Clinic showed that physician reduction in work effort was related to burnout and low satisfaction such that even a one-point increase in reported emotional exhaustion on a seven-point Likert scale was associated with 30%–40% increase in likelihood of reduced profes-sional effort in the next 24 months (Shanafelt et al. 2016b).

In addition, medical errors have financial costs and undermine the ethical and humanitarian goals of the organization. Medical errors have been tied to physician burnout across specialties, and the relationship is likely bidirectional (Tawfik et al. 2018). Physicians who experience burn-out are at greater risk of making medical errors, and physicians who have made medical errors may be particularly vulnerable to experiencing burn-out. Alameddine and colleagues (2009) have asserted that medical errors are often evidence of system failure, not individual clinician carelessness (Alameddine et al. 2009). Even small differences in burnout symptoms are associated with fewer medical errors, meaning that efforts to improve clinician engagement, even among staff who are not experiencing the full burnout syndrome, could potentially have meaningful effects on reducing errors (Tawfik et al. 2018).

Health care systems are increasingly monitoring physician distress as part of their global quality metrics (Wallace et al. 2009). Although there may be concern that improvements to physician well-being will cost too much to be realistic in a viable business model or will conflict with other organizational imperatives such as providing the highest quality of care, emerging evidence suggests that this is not the case. Greater physician engagement is good for business and quality of care, and many effective interventions add minimal additional cost to an organization's bottom line (Shanafelt and Noseworthy 2017).

The professional role of mental health care clinicians is to help patients enhance their own self-care and well-being. Physicians who take care of their own health also provide better screening and counseling about health practices to their own patients (Frank et al. 2000; Lewis et al. 1991). This fact is true across diverse health areas, including smoking cessation, nutrition, and exercise (Frank et al. 2010). As comprehensive health care systems move to population-based care and integrate prevention and wellness education for their patients as a strategy for reducing long-term health care costs, attention to the well-being of practicing clinicians has the potential to dually benefit both clinician and patient.

Variability Across Settings

The impact of systems issues and the opportunities for intervention vary significantly across settings where clinicians work. For instance, practice inefficiencies and clerical burden are universal contributors to clinician burnout, but the way they manifest may be different across settings. Compensation structures also vary across settings. For some clinicians, earned income depends directly on productivity (Conrad et al. 2002). In other settings, clinicians are salaried and may or may not have opportunities for bonuses or advancement based on strong productivity (Khullar et al. 2015; Robinson et al. 2004). Each structure has diverse consequences for physician engagement and burnout (Dyrbye et al. 2017).

In spite of this substantial variability across specialties, professionals providing direct patient care are at highest risk of burnout (Panagioti et al. 2017; Shanafelt et al. 2012a). The emotional toll of mental health care, combined with the increasing demands for clinical productivity across many organization types, make clinicians particularly vulnerable. In academic medical centers, where faculty may also be committed to educational and scientific missions, these forces may place strain on faculty members who would find their best career fit engaging in more teaching or research (Shanafelt et al. 2009).

Clearly defined job descriptions for hiring are critical to achieving alignment between job demands and an individual's professional values and career ambitions. When clinicians find themselves in a position where organizational priorities are out of sync with their own sense of professional contribution or meaning, burnout is likely (Shanafelt et al. 2009, 2016a). Table 6–2 provides some examples of the unique challenges and opportunities posed by several common employment settings.

Tiered Primary Prevention as a Model for System-Level Intervention

In large health care systems with many clinicians, the task of providing tailored services to professionals with a wide range of potential needs is daunting. For this reason, many systems have begun to use a tiered primary prevention model (Chaukos et al. 2018). Systems can be developed for preventing clinician burnout from developing (tier I), identifying and supporting individuals at particular risk (tier II), and providing focused intervention options for people who are already experiencing adverse effects (tier III). This type of model as shown in Figure 6–1 can be a helpful way to conceptualize the critical goals of prevention, screening, and treatment at both individual and system levels.

In the tiered model, prevention efforts are aimed at the whole workforce. Efforts include basic training related to wellness practices, supports for clinician self-care, and assisting clinicians in doing meaningful work and balancing personal responsibilities. Prevention strategies are also being applied in training programs to support student mental health. For instance, as part of a comprehensive medical student wellness program, Vanderbilt's School of Medicine has begun to integrate well-being topics directly into the curriculum (Drolet and Rodgers 2010).

TABLE 6–2. Challenges and opportunities in clinician wellness across settings

Setting	Challenges for clinician wellness	Opportunities
Private practice	• Potential for isolation from colleagues • Clinicians responsible for many administrative tasks • Salaries often directly linked to clinical revenue	• High levels of autonomy to determine schedule and other characteristics of the practice
Primary care	• Isolation from other mental health professionals • Scope of practice opportunities possibly limited by managed care	• Support from colleagues from other disciplines • Greater patient access to system of care
Hospital system	• Fast-paced work environment • Decreased autonomy of clinicians • Clerical burden • Clinicians at all levels of training	• Availability of comprehensive benefit packages and employee wellness programs
Public schools	• Isolation from other mental health professionals • Available resources strained due to legal obligation to comply with Individualized Education Plan	• Access to school staff who observe patients daily • Work schedule aligned with public school calendar
U.S. Department of Veterans Affairs	• Acuity of patient population	• Large network of clinicians and care systems
Community mental health	• Limited resources of clinics • Patients who may be living in poverty or have significant financial stressors	• Colleagues who likely share passion for helping underserved patients • Potential for creative program development to have tremendous impact

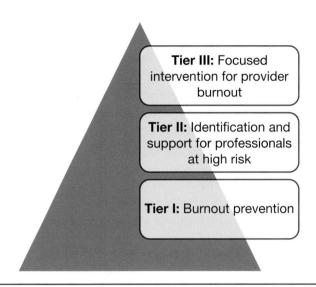

FIGURE 6–1. Tiered primary prevention model for addressing clinician burnout.

Monitoring programs are also an important part of prevention efforts in that any clinician who may be experiencing outsized distress can be identified for further supports (tiers II and III). Measurement is key for this strategy to work (Linzer et al. 2014; Wallace et al. 2009). Although health care systems routinely monitor patient volume, revenue, safety, and satisfaction, data are not always readily available regarding the health and well-being of clinicians. Given how critical a healthy workforce is to both quality of care and organizational viability long term, adoption of a routine practice of assessing clinician wellness as part of institutional performance is recommended. A variety of useful measures are readily available for this purpose, including national benchmark data to aid interpretation (Dyrbye et al. 2016; Shanafelt and Noseworthy 2017; Shanafelt et al. 2012a, 2015b). Once clinicians who are at risk for or already experiencing burnout are identified, supports or targeted interventions can be provided.

Common Structures for Supporting Clinician Wellness

Strategies commonly employed to support clinician wellness can involve management practices, professional development opportunities, and specific benefit packages. For instance, The Joint Commission currently requires hospitals to have a program to encourage physician wellness. Large health care systems have greater capacity to offer many of these services. In small practices, innovative approaches are likely needed to provide comparable benefits.

The first category of supports for clinician wellness relates directly to the nature of the work. Reasonable work demands and a manageable schedule are critical components of sustainable practice. Long hours and heavy documentation burden appear to have more negative influence on well-being than number of patients, suggesting that workplace efficiencies have the potential to reduce burnout (Rupert et al. 2015). Lack of control over work schedule appears to be a particularly significant contributor to risk for burnout. Flexibility in allowing clinicians to tailor their work effort and hours to meet both personal and professional obligations can prevent or help clinicians recover from burnout (Mechaber et al. 2008; Shanafelt et al. 2016b). Flexible scheduling has also been suggested as a way to allow clinicians to meet both personal and professional obligations without reducing work effort (Shanafelt and Noseworthy 2017). Depending on personal circumstances, working some longer days and some shorter days or pushing back start time for clinic activities may be viable options that work well for clinicians and patients. Giving employees control over the nature of their work is also a powerful intervention (Dyrbye et al. 2017; Williams et al. 2002).

Another aspect of professional wellness relates to professional growth and career development. Mentorship structures support employees so they can make meaningful contributions in their field and advance in their careers. Access to several mentors who each serves a distinct role, sometimes termed *mosaic mentoring*, as discussed in Chapter 2, "Professional and Personal Developmental Milestones," can be optimal. In academic medicine, mentorship may have a particularly powerful effect on the productivity and professional advancement of women and minorities (Beech et al. 2013; Benson et al. 2002; McGuire et al. 2004; Welch et al. 2012; Zisook and Dunn 2013).

The final category relates to personal issues. The long hours associated with a full-time position in medicine or mental health care can make it difficult to attend to necessary personal and family responsibilities. Cultural and societal expectations around caregiving can be particularly strong for women, which can exacerbate this challenge (Dyrbye et al. 2011, 2012; Shanafelt and Noseworthy 2017). The reality is that many employees will experience personal or family situations requiring a leave from work. Clear communication about state laws, company practice governing leaves of absence, and processes for accessing employee assistance programs is foundational. Employees need clear guidance regarding paid time off. Some workplaces have a mechanism for employees to access counseling services if needed. Access to resources, such as childcare, back-up care, employee support groups, or healthy living classes, can also support employee wellness. Other workplaces offer access to food, rest areas, or exercise facilities, which employees can use during the workday. Workplace culture must also support and align with policies regarding leave and benefits. Disincentives for taking earned vacation time, for instance, whether formal or informal, will likely undermine workforce motivation and productivity.

Emerging Program Models

Several health care systems have developed comprehensive physician wellness programs that serve as models for other organizations. Certainly, each system faces challenges unique to its own workforce, patient population, community resources, and other factors. Nevertheless, it can be helpful to review examples of how a system could implement a package of multifaceted supports. Several of these models are focused on medicine and physicians in particular, but many of the supports are applicable to psychiatry, psychology, and mental health care.

Shanafelt and Noseworthy (2017) outlined nine organizational strategies to promote physician engagement supported by both the growing body of literature on the topic and their own experiences. They argued that organizational commitment to reducing burnout can make a difference if comprehensive and sustained efforts are employed. They explained that even relatively inexpensive investments can have broad impact, especially if the program is championed by executive leadership.

In 2007, the Mayo Clinic launched a program on physician well-being focused on the dual goals of improving wellness in their workforce and advancing the science related to system-level interventions to combat burnout and increase engagement. The program has become a highly respected model because of its success in bringing physician burnout in line with, and in some cases below, national benchmarks (Shanafelt et al. 2012a, 2015a), even while the system also implemented familiar programs to increase efficiency, decrease costs, and increase productivity. Rates of burnout for nonphysician employees also declined during the same period.

Several other institutions across the country have begun to develop comprehensive models for supporting physician well-being. For instance, Vanderbilt's School of Medicine has developed a comprehensive medical student wellness program with a well-being curriculum to enhance the personal development of physicians-in-training (Drolet and Rodgers 2010). The School of Medicine at University of California, Davis, has also implemented a comprehensive program focused on supporting physician well-being, which includes prevention activities; a mechanism for physicians experiencing burnout or psychiatric symptoms to access clinical care; and educational activities for students, faculty, and their family members (Seritan et al. 2015). The University of California has also made a deliberate effort to institute family-friendly employment policies (available on its website at https://www.ucop.edu/faculty-diversity/policies-guidelines/family-friendly-practices-and-policies/family-friendly-policies-and-issues.html replacement).

Another model is emerging in the newly established Stanford University School of Medicine's WellMD Center (see https://wellmd.stanford.edu). The program represents a major institutional investment in clinician well-being across the School of Medicine and the university's two hospital systems. The program has the goal of creating programs to enhance personal resilience, as well as improve efficiency of practice and establish an organizational culture of wellness.

Many other programs are already under way or under development. A wealth of information regarding best practices should soon emerge as a result of widespread implementation of wellness programs.

Importance of Clinician Involvement in Wellness Initiatives

Although senior leadership support for system-wide interventions is important, a case can also be made for grassroots efforts driven by the desires of practicing mental health clinicians themselves. Some of the power of stakeholder involvement comes from the fact that having control over one's work environment is itself a key antidote to burnout. For this reason alone, involving clinicians at all levels in workplace decisions will itself reduce burnout to some extent. Even if the first interventions tried are not immediately successful, the process can create a sense of employee engagement, and the team can work together to develop and test the next intervention option (Shanafelt and Noseworthy 2017). All theories about drivers of professional burnout acknowledge the key role of a professional's sense of control over work. For instance, Maslach proposed six work environment characteristics that are important conditions for employee engagement: control, workload, community, rewards, fairness, and values (Maslach et al. 2001). Other models have highlighted similar factors, including status, certainty, autonomy, relatedness, and fairness (Tillott et al. 2013). When compared with externally mandated changes, interventions or supports derived from the local work environment may more directly increase a physician's sense of control and engagement (West et al. 2016).

In response to the recognized benefits of local work initiatives, the Mayo Clinic recently reported on the Listen-Act-Develop model for physician-organization collaboration to support wellness (Swensen et al. 2016). The model recognizes that empowering clinicians to contribute to the wellness solutions can likely enhance control, autonomy, and overall well-being far more than anything an administrator or executive could mandate or change alone. The more empowered employees feel to suggest enhancements to the work environment, the more professionally engaged they will be.

The sense an individual employee has about his or her job's meaning and the employee's ability to influence outcomes have been termed *psychological empowerment* (Spreitzer 1995). Employees who feel empowered are typically more engaged in their jobs and committed to the organization (Ahmad and Oranye 2010). Organizational research has increasingly acknowledged the critical role of psychological empowerment in successful service-oriented workplaces, including health care organizations. For instance, a study of nurses in China identified the importance of balancing job demands with opportunities for participating in decision-making and governance in order to enhance employee psychological empowerment (Fan et al. 2016).

A participatory management style with collaborative action planning has been suggested for engaging employees in identifying local factors to improve satisfaction and reduce burnout (Shanafelt and Noseworthy 2017). When leaders acknowledge the critical roles employees play in informing and tailoring effective workplace interventions, leaders enhance the sense of empowerment and control in the workforce. Many of the characteristics that make a good physician or mental health professional, such as critical thinking, data-based decision-making, empathy, and the ability to evaluate and develop solutions to complex problems, also mean that these employees have unique and valuable strengths to contribute to ensuring organizational health and building an engaging work culture.

Success Stories From Implementation of Novel Support Measures

Although high job demands contribute to burnout, recent evidence in-dicates that applying alternative resources to counteract these forces, such as professional development opportunities, feedback, and mentor-ship (Rupert et al. 2015), may be quite effective. In an effort to improve clinician wellness, many innovative strategies are being tried. Beyond schedule adjustments or workload reduction, these strategies often aim to change the organizational culture, improve teamwork and meaning-ful supervision, and increase employee agency (Panagioti et al. 2017).

The greatest evidence for organizational-level modifications for phy-sicians comes from studies of work hour restrictions (West et al. 2016), such as rotating on-duty and off-duty periods, separating day and night shift assignments, modifications to clinical work processes, shortened resident shifts, and protected time for interns to sleep (Ali et al. 2011; Garland et al. 2012; Panagioti et al. 2017). In recognition of the impor-tance of this issue, the Accreditation Council for Graduate Medical Ed-ucation now mandates sleep deprivation education for residents and has implemented duty hour restrictions. Other types of grading modifi-cations and curricular changes are also being attempted in medical schools, in recognition of the idea that some of the historically distress-ing and "cutthroat" aspects of medical education are not necessary to accomplish effective training (Moir et al. 2018; Slavin et al. 2014).

In keeping with the goal of giving clinicians sustainable workloads, many health care systems are experimenting with different ways to re-duce the burden of documentation on clinicians. Evidence suggests that doctors spend less time providing patient care and more time docu-menting care and that the near-universal adoption of EHRs has brought with it increased expectations for documentation and correspondence. Better measurement of the problem is one key to developing solutions. DiAngi and colleagues (2017) have proposed novel metrics (e.g., how fre-quently employees complete documentation during nights and week-ends or "work after work") for capturing EHR burden. Systems of scribes to draft documentation for doctors to review are also being piloted, with promising initial results in terms of physician satisfaction (Gidwani et al. 2017; Sharp and Stevens 2019).

Innovative compensation structures are likely needed to support both productivity and wellness (Shanafelt and Noseworthy 2017). For in-stance, simply compensating clinicians financially for productivity may incentivize overwork and fuel feelings of burnout. As health care systems transition to value-based purchasing, organizations are also likely to transition compensation models to align with quality of performance rather than solely volume-based compensation (Khullar et al. 2015). Compensation based on quality indicators is not always more effective (Gavagan et al. 2010; Rosenthal and Frank 2006). Centers have begun to experiment with compensation models to incorporate aspects of self-care and well-being in the calculations of productivity-based pay (Shanafelt and Noseworthy 2017). By rewarding productive clinicians with protected time to pursue meaningful scholarly or programmatic projects or by incorporating greater schedule flexibility, it is possible to contribute to higher feelings of professional fulfillment and less conflict in work-life integration.

A variety of other technology-based solutions are also being proposed. For instance, applications that allow clinicians to access critical patient care data remotely give clinicians greater flexibility in work location. Technology can also enhance scheduling flexibility. The increasing acceptance of telehealth solutions will allow clinicians more flexibility in providing patient care remotely. Telehealth has also been proposed as a way for clinicians to access confidential mental health care for themselves when needed, bypassing the confidentiality issues inherent when a clinician needs care provided within the system where the clinician already works.

Workplace spaces can also be designed to foster community and interaction among physicians. Pressure to use all available space for patient care can lead many institutions to eliminate lounges and meeting areas. By contrast, the Mayo Clinic has implemented several deliberate strategies for promoting community (Shanafelt and Noseworthy 2017). These strategies include designating meeting areas with workstations and healthy food options and using the resulting emergence of space to promote camaraderie and interaction among physicians, researchers, and administrators across several of their campuses. Employee engagement in quality improvement projects designed to improve communication or workflow may also yield beneficial effects (Linzer et al. 2015; Panagioti et al. 2017). Other approaches have included gathering clinicians together for discussion, such as in Doctoring to Heal or Balint groups that were designed to enhance personal awareness and explore physician-patient relationships, respectively (Epstein 1999; Rabow and McPhee 2001; West et al. 2014).

In another example, providing physicians with 1 hour of protected time every other week to meet with colleagues and discuss topics related to professional roles was found to improve physicians' sense of meaning and reduce burnout (West et al. 2014). Specifically, the intervention involved facilitated biweekly meetings for physicians, which were designed to enhance collegiality and community by incorporating aspects of mindfulness, shared experience, and reflection into a small-group discussion. Physicians who engaged in these discussion groups showed significant improvement in depersonalization, emotional exhaustion, and overall burnout, as well as greater empowerment, engagement, and ratings of their work's meaningfulness. The control group also received protected time but did not participate in the group meetings and in functioning during the study period.

A follow-up study of Colleagues Meeting to Promote and Sustain Satisfaction (COMPASS) groups provided a more scalable model in which physicians meet to share a meal every 2 weeks with a group of six to seven colleagues (West et al. 2015). The first 20 minutes of the gathering are spent discussing a question that explores the challenges and virtues of being a physician. The cost of the meal ($20 per person) was supported by the institution and is substantially lower than the cost of the protected time model.

Practical support for personal obligations is another innovative approach to assist busy clinicians with integrating meaningful work into a fulfilling personal life. For instance, a pilot program in the Emergency Medicine Department at Stanford University compensated physicians who volunteered for extra shifts or committee work with credits for prepared family meals or household help (Fassiotto et al. 2018).

Other efforts have been focused on helping clinicians to engage in meaningful work and achieve greater professional fulfillment. For instance, one suggested solution involves designing a clinician's schedule so that the clinician devotes at least 20% of his or her time to care in an area that has personal meaning for him or her. Evidence from a survey of internal medicine faculty suggested that this practice could dramatically reduce the risk of burnout (Shanafelt et al. 2009). Innovative mentorship and professional coaching programs are also emerging, based on the rationale that if clinicians receive coaching to improve leadership effectiveness, they will experience greater professional engagement and fulfillment (Frich et al. 2015). Evidence suggests that for early-career professionals or clinicians who care for particularly complex patient populations, interventions that are focused on teamwork, mentoring, and leadership skill development may be particularly impactful (Panagioti et al. 2017).

In recognition of the fact that cultivating a workforce of engaged professionals requires substantial leadership skill, other systems are piloting leadership training programs that can assess the extent to which senior leaders are effective at fostering a healthy work culture and provide targeted interventions to improve leadership effectiveness (McCallister and Hamilton 2019). Supporting leaders in fostering alignment of core values among staff can be particularly powerful. Clearly, supervisor behavior has substantial effects on the wellness of the clinicians they supervise (Shanafelt et al. 2015a; Williams et al. 2007). These priorities must be taken into account in hiring senior administrators, assessing their effectiveness, providing regular feedback, and coaching to support leadership development. Decisions about when to retain and promote leaders and when to make leadership changes to better support treatment teams and programs can also be important.

Need for System-Level Change

Increasingly, there have been calls for a major overhaul of specific aspects of health care systems that consistently undermine both patient care and clinician well-being. For instance, the documentation required for billing clinical encounters has been criticized for being minimally related to safety or quality of care and unsustainable for clinicians. Significant streamlining is needed, as well as acknowledgment that many tasks restricted to attendings can be safely and effectively performed by other members of the health care team (Shanafelt and Noseworthy 2017). Input from a wide range of stakeholders will be needed to develop workable systems.

Another concern often raised is the issue of maintenance of certification and medical licensure and continuing education. When clinicians are required to self-disclose all diagnoses or treatment for mental health conditions during licensing, they may fear that approval depends on having a record free from any mental health care. This system unfortunately can discourage students and practicing professionals from seeking help they may need to practice effectively (Shanafelt and Noseworthy 2017). Evidence suggests that even when physicians experience serious psychiatric symptoms, few may seek care (Shanafelt et al. 2011a). Although current impairment is highly relevant to a professional's fitness for practice, a historical diagnosis or evidence of a treatment history is less clearly relevant to patient safety. The goal should be to have a system that can balance public safety with fair treatment for physicians who may need care but can still practice safely (Seritan 2013).

Advancing the Science of Professional Wellness

Organizational supports may even enhance the effectiveness of interventions directed at individual clinicians (Panagioti et al. 2017; West et al. 2014). In addition, advancing organizational science is essential so that new knowledge is created to promote greater engagement among future generations of clinicians. Existing evidence suggests that combinations of structural changes, communication interventions, and cultivation of teamwork may be most effective at reducing burnout (Swensen et al. 2016). There are a limited number of controlled trials addressing organizational supports for burnout prevention and intervention. This issue should be regarded as a funding priority given its widespread implications for population health (Dyrbye et al. 2017; Shanafelt et al. 2017).

Although important scientific questions can be methodologically challenging to address, recent research has revealed increasing commitment to the investigation of meaningful and valued workplace practices. Better measurement tools will also substantially aid the advancing science of professional wellness, and these must continue to be developed and refined. Brady et al. (2018) argue the need for greater consistency in definition of physician wellness and measurement of this important construct across studies. Measurement of positive factors related to well-being, such as professional fulfillment, in addition to assessment of burnout, is particularly important (Trockel et al. 2018). Innovative measurement within health care systems, potentially even using EHR-based data analytics, can also help systems measure factors that reflect the institution's and clinicians' true goals and help systems change when goals or core values are misaligned (DiAngi et al. 2017). Other types of emerging technologies, such as wearable devices capable of tracking activity and sleep patterns, may likely be used with increasing frequency in wellness programs (Chaukos et al. 2018) once methodological challenges are overcome.

More research is clearly needed to identify effective practices. For instance, although many studies have now been published on interventions to reduce physician burnout, the majority have had methodological limitations (Baker and Sen 2016; Regehr et al. 2014). There is still limited information about which practices are likely to work best for certain subgroups of clinicians and how individual and system-level interventions can be optimally combined (West et al. 2016). Measures of burnout are widely used, and measures of professional fulfillment are emerging. In particular, systems that are functioning well will need to be carefully examined. In addition, improved measurement of optimal outcomes at both the clinician level and the system level are critically needed. Further studies, particularly of model systems with high levels of physician engagement, are likely to yield great insight and future benefit.

A cultural shift is occurring in which people are beginning to acknowledge and value clinician wellness. Coordinated effort among stakeholders at national and local levels is likely needed for substantive progress (Shanafelt et al. 2017). The increased scientific attention to this important issue provides substantial hope. The more serious scientific and political attention is placed on solving this problem, the more clinicians, patients, and the public will benefit.

Positive Practices

The following are several specific positive practices that readers are encouraged to try for themselves.

1. Take time to reflect on which aspects of your work are the most personally meaningful to you. Do you most value time with patients? Clinical or classroom teaching? Advancing research? New program development? Leadership and administrative roles? If you are spending less than 1 day per week in the activity that has the most meaning for you, set a goal to increase this (even by an hour or two at first). If you work in a setting where you have limited control over your own schedule, it may take time to adjust the balance of your work assignments. Make sure those you work with and for are aware of your passion and enlist their support. Risk of burnout may be almost double for those professionals who spend less than 10% of their time on personally meaningful types of work.

2. Find a way to give clinicians you supervise more control over their own work. Is there a decision you need to make for which you could solicit input from employees to guide your choice? Is there a way to offer a more flexible work schedule? When launching a new project, can you ask multiple staff members who might be involved and take volunteers instead of just assigning a staff person yourself? Full autonomy is almost never possible in health care systems, but when professionals feel they have control over aspects of their work life and choices about when and how to work, well-being is enhanced.

3. Emerging evidence suggests that even 1 hour every other week to discuss professional issues with colleagues can have substantial well-

being benefit. If weekly or biweekly meetings are too difficult to schedule, try a monthly dinner, lunch, or breakfast. Use this time to give and
receive support from colleagues, acknowledge the reality of work challenges, and explicitly discuss together what helps you fight burnout
and sustain passion for your work.

4. Show your colleagues that you value well-being by taking wellness
   into consideration in workplace decisions that are under your control. If you supervise trainees, uphold policies that support their
   health. If you are mentoring junior colleagues, explicitly acknowledge
   the challenges they may face in work-life integration and offer support and guidance based on your experience. If you have opportunities to take on leadership roles within your organization, use your
   influence to guide policy decisions that are consistent with wellness.

5. Learn about the available resources within your organization for
   burnout prevention, screening, and treatment. Participate in any surveys about wellness and answer honestly. If your organization has a
   program to enhance well-being, find a way to get involved. For many
   professionals, finding a way to help others feel more satisfied with
   their work can be satisfying in return.

Conclusion

System-level commitment to wellness is a viable business practice with
potential for substantial benefit to both clinicians and patients in the
short and long term. A growing body of research brings substantial hope
that this science will continue to grow and inform clinical and business
practices. Balancing professional autonomy with alignment on core values and support for professional development across the organization is
key. Cooperation across a diverse set of individual, organizational, and
governmental stakeholders will be necessary. When clinicians feel that
their contributions are valued, that their choices are respected, and that
they have opportunities for growth and meaningful contribution, they
and the systems in which they work will benefit.

Questions to Discuss With Colleagues and Mentors
———————o———————

- What is the impact of clinician burnout in the workplace? Does
  burnout contribute to clinician turnover in our clinic?

- What tiered strategies for preventing burnout are possible at work?
- What can we do to strengthen clinician engagement in the workplace setting?
- Compared with other places where you have worked, what does the current workplace do well? What could be done better?
- How does burnout relate to other kinds of workplace issues we face?

—————O—————

Recommended Resources

McCallister D, Hamilton T (eds): Transforming the Heart of Practice: An Organizational and Personal Approach to Physician Wellbeing. Cham, Switzerland, Springer, 2019

National Academy of Medicine: Organizational strategies. Washington, DC, National Academy of Medicine, 2019. Available at: https://nam.edu/clinicianwellbeing/solutions/organizational-strategies. Accessed August 11, 2019.

Panagioti M, Panagopoulou E, Bower P, et al: Controlled interventions to reduce burnout in physicians: a systematic review and meta-analysis. JAMA Intern Med 177(2):195–205, 2017

Roberts LW, Trockel MT (eds): The Art and Science of Physician Wellbeing: A Handbook for Physicians and Trainees. Cham, Switzerland, Springer, 2019

Shanafelt TD, Noseworthy JH: Executive leadership and physician wellbeing: nine organizational strategies to promote engagement and reduce burnout. Mayo Clin Proc 92(1):129–146, 2017

Sotile WM, Sotile MO: The Resilient Physician: Effective Emotional Management for Doctors and Their Medical Organizations. Chicago, IL, American Medical Association, 2002

Walton GM, Brady ST: The many questions of belonging, in Handbook of Competence and Motivation: Theory and Application, 2nd Edition. Edited by Elliott AJ, Dweck CS, Yeager DS. New York, Guilford, 2018, pp 272–293

West CP, Dyrbye LN, Rabatin JT, et al: Intervention to promote physician wellbeing, job satisfaction, and professionalism: a randomized clinical trial. JAMA Intern Med 174(4):527–533, 2014

References

Ahmad N, Oranye NO: Empowerment, job satisfaction and organizational commitment: a comparative analysis of nurses working in Malaysia and England. J Nurs Manag 18(5):582–591, 2010 20636507

Alameddine M, Dainty KN, Deber R, Sibbald WJ: The intensive care unit work environment: current challenges and recommendations for the future. J Crit Care 24(2):243–248, 2009 19327295

Ali NA, Hammersley J, Hoffmann SP, et al: Continuity of care in intensive care units: a cluster-randomized trial of intensivist staffing. Am J Respir Crit Care Med 184(7):803–808, 2011 21719756

Awa WL, Plaumann M, Walter U: Burnout prevention: a review of intervention programs. Patient Educ Couns 78(2):184–190, 2010 19467822

Baker K, Sen S: Healing medicine's future: prioritizing physician trainee mental health. AMA J Ethics 18(6):604–613, 2016 27322994

Becher H, Dollard M: Psychosocial Safety Climate and Better Productivity in Australian Workplaces: Costs, Productivity, Presenteeism, Absenteeism. Canberra, Australia, Safe Work Australia, November 2016. Available at: www.safeworkaustralia.gov.au/system/files/documents/1705/psychosocial-safety-climate-and-better-productivity-in-australian-workplaces-nov-2016.pdf. Accessed August 11, 2019.

Beddoe AE, Murphy SO: Does mindfulness decrease stress and foster empathy among nursing students? J Nurs Educ 43(7):305–312, 2004 15303583

Beech BM, Calles-Escandon J, Hairston KG, et al: Mentoring programs for underrepresented minority faculty in academic medical centers: a systematic review of the literature. Acad Med 88(4):541–549, 2013 23425989

Benson CA, Morahan PS, Sachdeva AK, Richman RC: Effective faculty preceptoring and mentoring during reorganization of an academic medical center. Med Teach 24(5):550–557, 2002 12450479

Bodenheimer T, Sinsky C: From triple to quadruple aim: care of the patient requires care of the provider. Ann Fam Med 12(6):573–576, 2014 25384822

Brady KJS, Trockel MT, Khan CT, et al: What do we mean by physician wellness? A systematic review of its definition and measurement. Acad Psychiatry 42(1):94–108, 2018 28913621

Chaukos D, Vestal HS, Bernstein CA, et al: An ounce of prevention: a public health approach to improving physician well-being. Acad Psychiatry 42(1):150–154, 2018 28685352

Chung H, van der Horst M: Women's employment patterns after childbirth and the perceived access to and use of flexitime and teleworking. Hum Relat 71(1):47–72, 2018 29276304

Cimiotti J, Aiken L, Sloane D, Wu E: Nurse staffing, burnout, and health care-associated infection. Am J Infect Control 40(6):486–490, 2012 22854376

Conrad DA, Sales A, Liang S-Y, et al: The impact of financial incentives on physician productivity in medical groups. Health Serv Res, 37(4):885–906, 2002 12236389

Demerouti E, Bakker AB, Nachreiner F, Schaufeli WB: The job demands-resources model of burnout. J Appl Psychol 86(3):499–512, 2001 11419809

de Oliveira GS Jr, Chang R, Fitzgerald PC, et al: The prevalence of burnout and depression and their association with adherence to safety and practice standards: a survey of United States anesthesiology trainees. Anesth Analg 117(1):182–193, 2013 23687232

Dewa CS, Loong D, Bonato S, et al: How does burnout affect physician productivity? A systematic literature review. BMC Health Serv Res 14:325, 2014 25066375

DiAngi YT, Lee TC, Sinsky CA, et al: Novel metrics for improving professional fulfillment. Ann Intern Med 167(10):740–741, 2017 29052698

Drolet BC, Rodgers S: A comprehensive medical student wellness program—design and implementation at Vanderbilt School of Medicine. Acad Med 85(1):103–110, 2010 20042835

Dyrbye LN, Shanafelt TD, Balch CM, et al: Relationship between work-home conflicts and burnout among American surgeons: a comparison by sex. Arch Surg 146(2):211–217, 2011 21339435

Dyrbye LN, Freischlag J, Kaups KL, et al: Work-home conflicts have a substantial impact on career decisions that affect the adequacy of the surgical workforce. Arch Surg 147(10):933–939, 2012 23117833

Dyrbye LN, Satele D, Shanafelt T: Ability of a 9-item well-being index to identify distress and stratify quality of life in US workers. J Occup Environ Med 58(8):810–817, 2016 27294444

Dyrbye L, Shanafelt TD, Sinsky CA, et al: Burnout Among Health Care Professionals: A Call to Explore and Address This Underrecognized Threat to Safe, High-Quality Care. Washington, DC, National Academy of Medicine, July 5, 2017. Available at: https://nam.edu/wp-content/uploads/2017/07/Burnout-Among-Health-Care-Professionals-A-Call-to-Explore-and-Address-This-Underrecognized-Threat.pdf. Accessed August 11, 2019.

Enochs WK, Etzbach CA: Impaired student counselors: ethical and legal considerations for the family. Family Journal 12(4):396–400, 2004

Epstein RM: Mindful practice. JAMA 282(9):833–839, 1999 10478689

Fan Y, Zheng Q, Liu S, Li Q: Construction of a new model of job engagement, psychological empowerment and perceived work environment among Chinese registered nurses at four large university hospitals: implications for nurse managers seeking to enhance nursing retention and quality of care. J Nurs Manag 24(5):646–655, 2016 27039839

Fassiotto M, Simard C, Sandborg C, et al: An integrated career coaching and time-banking system promoting flexibility, wellness, and success: a pilot program at Stanford University School of Medicine. Acad Med 93(6):881–887, 2018 29298183

Firth-Cozens J, Greenhalgh J: Doctors' perceptions of the links between stress and lowered clinical care. Soc Sci Med 44(7):1017–1022, 1997 9089922

Frank E, Rothenberg R, Lewis C, Belodoff BF: Correlates of physicians' prevention-related practices: findings from the Women Physicians' Health Study. Arch Fam Med 9(4):359–367, 2000 10776365

Frank E, Segura C, Shen H, Oberg E: Predictors of Canadian physicians' prevention counseling practices. Can J Public Health 101(5):390–395, 2010 21214054

Frich JC, Brewster AL, Cherlin EJ, Bradley EH: Leadership development programs for physicians: a systematic review. J Gen Intern Med 30(5):656–674, 2015 25527339

Garland A, Roberts D, Graff L: Twenty-four-hour intensivist presence: a pilot study of effects on intensive care unit patients, families, doctors, and nurses. Am J Respir Crit Care Med 185(7):738–743, 2012 22246176

Gavagan TF, Du H, Saver BG, et al: Effect of financial incentives on improvement in medical quality indicators for primary care. J Am Board Fam Med 23(5):622–631, 2010 20823357

Gidwani R, Nguyen C, Kofoed A, et al: Impact of scribes on physician satisfaction, patient satisfaction, and charting efficiency: a randomized controlled trial. Ann Fam Med 15(5):427–433, 2017 28893812

Haas JS, Cook EF, Puopolo AL, et al: Is the professional satisfaction of general internists associated with patient satisfaction? J Gen Intern Med 15(2):122–128, 2000 10672116

Hall LH, Johnson J, Watt I, et al: Healthcare staff wellbeing, burnout, and patient safety: a systematic review. PLoS One 11(7):e0159015, 2016 27391946

Hamidi MS, Bohman B, Sandborg C, et al: Estimating institutional physician turnover attributable to self-reported burnout and associated financial burden: a case study. BMC Health Serv Res 18(1):851, 2018 30477483

Han S, Shanafelt TD, Sinsky CA, et al: Estimating the attributable cost of physician burnout in the United States. Ann Intern Med 170(11):784–790, 2019 31132791

Harris LM, Cumming SR, Campbell AJ: Stress and psychological well-being among allied health professionals. J Allied Health 35(4):198–207, 2006 17243434

Irving JA, Dobkin PL, Park J: Cultivating mindfulness in health care professionals: a review of empirical studies of mindfulness-based stress reduction (MBSR). Complement Ther Clin Pract 15(2):61–66, 2009 19341981

Khullar D, Kocher R, Conway P, Rajkumar R: How 10 leading health systems pay their doctors. Healthc (Amst) 3(2):60–62, 2015 26179724

Kirkland A: Critical perspectives on wellness. J Health Polit Policy Law 39(5):971–988, 2014 25037834

Konrad TR, Williams ES, Linzer M, et al: Measuring physician job satisfaction in a changing workplace and a challenging environment, SGIM Career Satisfaction Study Group, Society of General Internal Medicine. Med Care 37(11):1174–1182, 1999 10549620

Lee J, Lim N, Yang E, Lee SM: Antecedents and consequences of three dimensions of burnout in psychotherapists: a meta-analysis. Prof Psychol Res Pr 42(3):252–258, 2011

Lewis CE, Clancy C, Leake B, Schwartz JS: The counseling practices of internists. Ann Intern Med 114(1):54–58, 1991 1983933

Lim N, Kim EK, Kim H, et al: Individual and work-related factors influencing burnout of mental health professionals: a meta-analysis. J Employ Couns 47(2):86–96, 2010

Linzer M, Levine R, Meltzer D, et al: 10 bold steps to prevent burnout in general internal medicine. J Gen Intern Med 29(1):18–20, 2014 24002633

Linzer M, Poplau S, Grossman E, et al: A cluster randomized trial of interventions to improve work conditions and clinician burnout in primary care: results from the Healthy Work Place (HWP) study. J Gen Intern Med 30(8):1105–1111, 2015 25724571

LoboPrabhu S, Summers RF, Moffic HS (eds): Combating Physician Burnout: A Guide for Psychiatrists. Washington, DC, American Psychiatric Association Publishing, 2020

MacKinnon M, Murray S: Reframing physician burnout as an organizational problem: a novel pragmatic approach to physician burnout. Acad Psychiatry 42(1):123–128, 2018 28247366

Maslach C, Schaufeli WB, Leiter MP: Job burnout. Annu Rev Psychol 52:397–422, 2001 11148311

McCallister D, Hamilton T (eds): Transforming the Heart of Practice: An Organizational and Personal Approach to Physician Wellbeing. Cham, Switzerland, Springer, 2019

McGuire LK, Bergen MR, Polan ML: Career advancement for women faculty in a U.S. school of medicine: perceived needs. Acad Med 79(4):319–325, 2004 15044163

Mechaber HF, Levine RB, Manwell LB, et al: Part-time physicians…prevalent, connected, and satisfied. J Gen Intern Med 23(3):300–303, 2008 18214623

Moir F, Yielder J, Sanson J, Chen Y: Depression in medical students: current insights. Adv Med Educ Pract 9:323–333, 2018 29765261

Panagioti M, Panagopoulou E, Bower P, et al: Controlled interventions to reduce burnout in physicians: a systematic review and meta-analysis. JAMA Intern Med 177(2):195–205, 2017 27918798

Rabow MW, McPhee SJ: Doctoring to Heal: fostering well-being among physicians through personal reflection. West J Med 174(1):66–69, 2001 11154679

Regehr C, Glancy D, Pitts A, LeBlanc VR: Interventions to reduce the consequences of stress in physicians: a review and meta-analysis. J Nerv Ment Dis 202(5):353–359, 2014 24727721

Robinson JC, Shortell SM, Li R, et al: The alignment and blending of payment incentives within physician organizations. Health Serv Res 39(5):1589–1606, 2004 15333124

Rosenthal MB, Frank RG: What is the empirical basis for paying for quality in health care? Med Care Res Rev 63(2):135–157, 2006 16595409

Rupert PA, Miller AO, Dorociak KE: Preventing burnout: what does the research tell us? Prof Psychol Res Pr 46(3):168–174, 2015

Santos MC, Barros L, Carolino E: Occupational stress and coping resources in physiotherapists: a survey of physiotherapists in three general hospitals. Physiotherapy 96(4):303–310, 2010 21056165

Schaufeli WB, Leiter MP, Maslach C: Burnout: 35 years of research and practice. Career Development International 14(3):204–220, 2009

Scheurer D, McKean S, Miller J, Wetterneck T: U.S. physician satisfaction: a systematic review. J Hosp Med 4(9):560–568, 2009 20013859

Seritan AL: How to recognize and avoid burnout, in The Academic Medicine Handbook: A Guide to Achievement and Fulfillment for Academic Faculty. Edited by Roberts LW. New York, Springer, 2013, pp 447–453

Seritan AL, Rai G, Servis M, Pomeroy C: The office of student wellness: innovating to improve student mental health. Acad Psychiatry 39(1):80–84, 2015 24840666

Shanafelt TD: Enhancing meaning in work: a prescription for preventing physician burnout and promoting patient-centered care. JAMA 302(12):1338–1340, 2009 19773573

Shanafelt TD, Noseworthy JH: Executive leadership and physician well-being: nine organizational strategies to promote engagement and reduce burnout. Mayo Clin Proc 92(1):129–146, 2017 27871627

Shanafelt TD, Bradley KA, Wipf JE, Back AL: Burnout and self-reported patient care in an internal medicine residency program. Ann Intern Med 136(5):358–367, 2002 11874308

Shanafelt TD, West CP, Sloan JA, et al: Career fit and burnout among academic faculty. Arch Intern Med 169(10):990–995, 2009 19468093

Shanafelt TD, Balch CM, Bechamps G, et al: Burnout and medical errors among American surgeons. Ann Surg 251(6):995–1000, 2010 19934755

Shanafelt TD, Balch CM, Dyrbye L, et al: Special report: suicidal ideation among American surgeons. Arch Surg 146(1):54–62, 2011a 21242446

Shanafelt TD, Sloan J, Satele D, Balch C: Why do surgeons consider leaving practice? J Am Coll Surg 212(3): 421–422, 2011b 21356491

Shanafelt TD, Boone S, Tan L, et al: Burnout and satisfaction with work-life balance among US physicians relative to the general US population. Arch Intern Med 172(18):1377–1385, 2012a 22911330

Shanafelt TD, Oreskovich MR, Dyrbye LN, et al: Avoiding burnout: the personal health habits and wellness practices of US surgeons. Ann Surg 255(4):625–633, 2012b 22388107

Shanafelt TD, Raymond M, Kosty M, et al: Satisfaction with work-life balance and the career and retirement plans of US oncologists. J Clin Oncol 32(11):1127–1135, 2014 24616305

Shanafelt TD, Gorringe G, Menaker R, et al: Impact of organizational leadership on physician burnout and satisfaction. Mayo Clin Proc 90(4):432–440, 2015a 25796117

Shanafelt TD, Hasan O, Dyrbye LN, et al: Changes in burnout and satisfaction with work-life balance in physicians and the general US working population between 2011 and 2014. Mayo Clin Proc 90(12):1600–1613, 2015b 26653297

Shanafelt TD, Dyrbye LN, Sinsky C, et al: Relationship between clerical burden and characteristics of the electronic environment with physician burnout and professional satisfaction. Mayo Clin Proc 91(7):836–848, 2016a 27313121

Shanafelt TD, Mungo M, Schmitgen J, et al: Longitudinal study evaluating the association between physician burnout and changes in professional work effort. Mayo Clin Proc 91(4):422–431, 2016b 27046522

Shanafelt TD, Dyrbye LN, West CP: Addressing physician burnout: the way forward. JAMA 317(9):901–902, 2017 28196201

Sharp C, Stevens L: The electronic health record, in The Art and Science of Physician Wellbeing: A Handbook for Physicians and Trainees. Edited by Roberts LW, Trockel MT. Cham, Switzerland, Springer, 2019, pp 87–102

Sinsky C, Colligan L, Li L, et al: Allocation of physician time in ambulatory practice: a time and motion study in 4 specialties. Ann Intern Med 165(11):753–760, 2016 27595430

Skosnik PD, Chatterton RT Jr, Swisher T, Park S: Modulation of attentional inhibition by norepinephrine and cortisol after psychological stress. Int J Psychophysiol 36(1):59–68, 2000 10700623

Slavin SJ, Schindler DL, Chibnall JT: Medical student mental health 3.0: improving student wellness through curricular changes. Acad Med 89(4):573–577, 2014 24556765

Spreitzer GM: Psychological empowerment in the workplace: dimensions, measurement, and validation. Acad Manage J 38(5):1442–1465, 1995

Swensen S, Kabcenell A, Shanafelt T: Physician-organization collaboration reduces physician burnout and promotes engagement: the Mayo Clinic experience. J Healthc Manag 61(2):105–127, 2016 27111930

Tawfik DS, Sexton JB, Kan P, et al: Burnout in the neonatal intensive care unit and its relation to healthcare-associated infections. J Perinatol 37(3):315–320, 2017 27853320

Tawfik DS, Profit J, Morgenthaler TI, et al: Physician burnout, well-being, and work unit safety grades in relationship to reported medical errors. Mayo Clin Proc 93(11):1571–1580, 2018 30001832

Tillott S, Walsh K, Moxham L: Encouraging engagement at work to improve retention. Nurs Manag (Harrow) 19(10):27–31, 2013 23577562

Trockel M, Bohman B, Lesure E, et al: A brief instrument to assess both burnout and professional fulfillment in physicians: reliability and validity, including correlation with self-reported medical errors, in a sample of resident and practicing physicians. Acad Psychiatry 42(1):11–24 2018 29196982

Wallace JE, Lemaire JB, Ghali WA: Physician wellness: a missing quality indicator. Lancet 374(9702):1714–1721, 2009 19914516

Weinberg A, Creed F: Stress and psychiatric disorder in healthcare professionals and hospital staff. Lancet 355(9203):533–537, 2000 10683003

Welch JL, Jimenez HL, Walthall J, Allen SE: The women in emergency medicine mentoring program: an innovative approach to mentoring. J Grad Med Educ 4(3):362–366, 2012 23997883

Welp A, Meier LL, Manser T: Emotional exhaustion and workload predict clinician-rated and objective patient safety. Front Psychol 5:1573, 2015 25657627

West CP, Hauer KE: Reducing burnout in primary care: a step toward solutions. J Gen Intern Med 30(8):1056–1057, 2015 25910601

West CP, Huschka M, Novotny PJ, et al: Association of perceived medical errors with resident distress ad empathy: a prospective longitudinal study. JAMA 296(9):1071–1078, 2006 16954486

West CP, Tan AD, Habermann TM, et al: Association of resident fatigue and distress with perceived medical errors. JAMA 302(12):1294–1300, 2009 19773564

West CP, Dyrbye LN, Rabatin JT, et al: Intervention to promote physician well-being, job satisfaction, and professionalism: a randomized clinical trial. JAMA Intern Med 174(4):527–533, 2014 24515493

West CP, Dyrbye LN, Satele D, Shanafelt TD: A randomized controlled trial evaluating the effect of COMPASS (COlleagues Meeting to Promote and Sustain Satisfaction) small group sessions on physician well-being, meaning, and job satisfaction. J Gen Intern Med 30, S89, 2015

West CP, Dyrbye LN, Erwin PJ, Shanafelt TD: Interventions to prevent and reduce physician burnout: a systematic review and meta-analysis. Lancet 388(10057):2272–2281, 2016 27692469

Williams ES, Konrad TR, Linzer M, et al: Physician, practice, and patient characteristics related to primary care physician physical and mental health: results from the Physician Worklife Study. Health Serv Res 37(1):121–143, 2002 11949917

Williams ES, Manwell LB, Konrad TR, Linzer M: The relationship of organizational culture, stress, satisfaction, and burnout with physician-reported error and suboptimal patient care: results from the MEMO study. Health Care Manage Rev 32(3):203–212, 2007 17666991

Williams ES, Konrad TR, Scheckler WE, et al: Understanding physicians' intentions to withdraw from practice: the role of job satisfaction, job stress, mental and physical health. 2001. Health Care Manage Rev 35(2):105–115, 2010 20234217

Wise EH, Hersh MA, Gibson CM: Ethics, self-care and well-being for psychologists: reenvisioning the stress-distress continuum. Prof Psychol Res Pr 43(5):487–494, 2012

Zisook S, Dunn LB: How to build a national reputation for academic promotion, in The Academic Medicine Handbook: A Guide to Achievement and Fulfillment for Academic Faculty. Edited by Roberts LW. New York, Springer, 2013, pp 397–403

ༀ

CHAPTER 7

Legal and Ethical Issues in the Context of Impairment and Recovery

Mental health conditions, addiction, cognitive impairment, physical health issues, and other personal factors may lead to impairments that affect mental health professionals' behavior, judgment, and ability to practice competently and safely. When the personal well-being of mental health professionals and trainees is compromised to a severe degree, this represents a threat to the health and safety not only of the clinicians themselves but also of their patients. These professionals are granted special privileges and are entrusted by society with the well-being of patients. They are also expected to adhere to high standards and to participate in self-regulation, entailing important ethical and legal obligations.

Ethical and Legal Obligations

Ethical obligations are articulated by professional bodies, such as the American Psychiatric Association, the American Psychological Association, and the American Association for Marriage and Family Therapy, whereas legal obligations are governed by applicable state and federal laws. Clinicians need to be aware of both their ethical and their legal duties. These duties are overlapping, but not synonymous, as illustrated in Figure 7–1.

In either case, legal and ethical duties may lead to complex and difficult judgments about whether, when, what, and how to report a possibly impaired colleague. Medical professionals' views about reporting col-

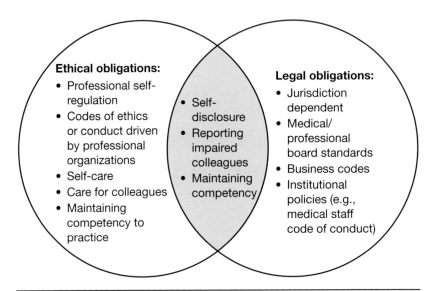

FIGURE 7–1.   Overlapping ethical and legal obligations related to clinician impairment.

leagues have been examined in several studies. For example, DesRoches and colleagues (2010) reported that although approximately two-thirds of physicians stated they felt "prepared" to report impaired or incompetent colleagues to authorities, several barriers stood in the way of reporting. Such barriers included worries about retribution, beliefs that nothing would result from reporting, and assumptions about someone else dealing with the issue. Being in a solo or two-person practice may have also been a factor in not reporting an impaired colleague, a finding that may have particular relevance for mental health professionals. Although the authors of this study argued that their findings suggested "a need for stronger external regulation" (p. 192), this view is controversial. Wynia (2010) argued that the findings suggest a need for further education of physicians in the basic tenets of professionalism (including self-regulation) and enhanced protections for the individuals who do report to reduce fear of retribution.

In this chapter, we include four in-depth case examples that illustrate a range of legal and ethical issues related to the competent practice of psychiatry and psychology and the obligations mental health professionals face in maintaining their own competence and supporting the competence of colleagues.

Case Example 1

Jake Pearson, Manuel Rio, and Daniel Singh are the only three psychiatrists who work in a suburban outpatient office that is operated by West-Care, a large, vertically integrated health care system. Drs. Rio and Singh are close friends, having worked together for more than 7 years. Dr. Pearson joined them 2 years ago, after retiring from solo practice in a town about 30 miles away. He had explained that he was tired of the hassles of running his own practice. Prior to hiring Dr. Pearson, WestCare had the position posted for 2 years, with no applicants. At WestCare, Dr. Pearson has minimal control of his schedule because the organization schedules patients (every 30 minutes) and works to minimize "blank space" (i.e., time without patients scheduled). The organization provides administrative time one afternoon per week for the psychiatrists to catch up on patient care–related tasks. Dr. Pearson, who previously kept paper charts at his private practice, must now learn how to use the organization's electronic medical record (EMR).

Dr. Pearson is rather private and talks only minimally with his colleagues when they see each other in the halls. On several occasions, he has mentioned his struggles with the EMR and seems frustrated that he is having trouble learning to use it efficiently. Although the three psychiatrists do not have regular team meetings, Drs. Rio and Singh frequently have lunch together and talk about patient care, their families, and music. Although they invite Dr. Pearson to join them, he never does and stays in his office "to catch up on these damn charts." Dr. Rio remarks to Dr. Singh, "It is almost as if he is still in private practice." They realize they do not even know if Dr. Pearson has a family or what he likes to do outside of work. On several occasions in the first 6 months after Dr. Pearson joined WestCare, Drs. Rio and Singh invited him to join them at a nearby restaurant after work for happy hour in an effort to help him feel more comfortable. Dr. Pearson declined each time, saying he had a long drive and wanted to get home "to take care of stuff." Eventually, Drs. Rio and Singh stopped inviting him and resigned themselves to a minimal relationship with their elusive colleague.

In the last 2 months, Dr. Pearson has arrived nearly an hour late on six occasions. Each time, he tells the clinic manager that he used to start later in private practice and is still getting used to the schedule. In addition, he has called in sick at least 1 day per week, leading to canceled patient visits and a significant amount of rescheduling. Three patients, who have had multiple appointments canceled, have asked to be reassigned to a different psychiatrist. Dr. Pearson does not say anything to his colleagues about what is happening and remains private. Concerned as well as frustrated, Drs. Rio and Singh ask him if there is something they can do to be of help. He responds by saying, "Thanks, but I think I'm getting better. I just can't seem to shake this cold."

Over the course of the next month, on the few occasions that he sees Dr. Pearson in the halls, Dr. Rio notices that his hands are shaky, and he appears sweaty. Dr. Rio decides to talk to Dr. Singh about the situation because he is concerned that Dr. Pearson's behavior could be explained by an alcohol use disorder. Drs. Rio and Singh discuss whether it is their role to confront their colleague or intervene in another way. They also wonder if they are ethically or legally obligated to report their colleague, how to report him, and to whom.

Although they want to do the right thing and are concerned about Dr. Pearson's health as well as the quality and continuity of care that his patients are receiving, they know they will have to absorb Dr. Pearson's patient panel if he leaves. They are also worried that it may be very difficult to find a replacement, given the shortage of psychiatrists in the area.

This scenario raises several dilemmas related to intervening with or reporting a potentially impaired colleague. Factors that may facilitate or hinder professionals' willingness to intervene with or report a possibly impaired colleague encompass several domains (Table 7–1), including psychological factors, professional or environmental factors (i.e., the work milieu or team dynamics), ethical factors, and legal or regulatory factors.

Drs. Rio and Singh are experiencing a number of these factors simultaneously, contributing to the challenge of determining next steps. From an ethical perspective, Drs. Rio and Singh have an obligation to intervene. The ethics codes of both the American Medical Association and the American Psychiatric Association emphasize the responsibility of physicians to intervene and to report and assist impaired colleagues. The codes do not prescribe specific actions for specific situations, however. Rather, they recognize the reality that every situation is unique. The American Psychiatric Association's Commentary on Ethics in Practice (available at www.psychiatry.org/psychiatrists/practice/ethics) explicitly notes that psychiatrists who are concerned about a colleague "may attempt to counsel or encourage the impaired colleague to seek treatment and to refrain from patient care."

In the case of Dr. Pearson, an initial consideration for Drs. Rio and Singh may be to seek consultation from a trusted colleague and to research what resources may be available for a local or regional physician health program. With such information in hand, when they do raise concerns with Dr. Pearson, they will be able to offer specific support to their colleague. If Dr. Pearson is unwilling to engage in a discussion of the issues, his colleagues will need to inform the physician well-being committee (or other institutional committee responsible for such instances).

One of the critical concerns of Dr. Pearson's colleagues is whether they should talk directly to Dr. Pearson or should report him to a pro-

TABLE 7–1. Factors that may affect professionals' willingness to intervene or report a potentially impaired colleague

Domain	Facilitators	Barriers
Psychological factors	• Desire to help colleague • Social bonds • Empathy • Personal or family history of psychiatric condition or addiction	• Fear of retaliation • Fear of increased burden • Fear of being sued • Personal situation (one's own stress or burnout) • Worry about one's own reputation
Professional or environmental factors	• High level of professionalism • Desire to protect patients • Team that functions well together and supports and trusts one another • Leadership that facilitates intervention	• Reduced professionalism • Worry about reflection on the field • Leadership that discourages intervention
Ethical factors	• Awareness of ethical obligation to intervene • Knowledge of profession's code of ethics	• Belief that it may be unethical if it may harm colleague • Vague, difficult-to-interpret ethics code
Legal or regulatory factors	• Awareness of state laws and medical or licensing board policies • Understanding of institutional or system policies	• Lack of awareness of reporting laws • Prior negative experience with reporting or with licensing board

gram or other body that would then take further action. In many cases, talking directly to the colleague would be preferable because this interaction may help the individual seek or accept treatment voluntarily. As illustrated in Table 7–2, the suspicions about Dr. Pearson's alcohol use disorder may be supported by the numerous signs he shows at work. It is also not the place of Dr. Pearson's colleagues to make a diagnosis, but rather they should encourage him to obtain appropriate evaluation and assistance.

A challenging issue in this case—as in many cases—is determining whether the individual is *impaired* because of his or her illness or addiction. According to the Federation of State Physician Health Programs (FSPHP; see www.fsphp.org/assets/docs/illness_vs_impairment.pdf), impairment should be distinguished from illness, although this distinction is not always the case with regulatory bodies.

The ability to seek help through a confidential process would almost certainly be preferable in cases like that of Dr. Pearson. The availability of voluntary options for seeking help, with appropriate monitoring to detect noncompliance or relapse, is likely responsible for the successful recovery of many physicians. A variety of programs are available for physicians with substance use disorders. In most states, there are funded, independent physician health programs (PHPs) that run assessment and monitoring programs. In other states that do not have their own PHPs, health systems take on the assessment and monitoring functions through physician well-being committees. The FSPHP was established to provide education and guidance to state PHPs, with the goal of assisting (rather than disciplining) impaired physicians, restoring health, and protecting patients.

Fortunately, the majority of physicians who enter substance abuse treatment programs do well in recovery and are able to maintain or return to practice. Psychiatrists appear to benefit from treatment as much as other physicians. For example, in a study by Yellowlees and colleagues (2014), among a longitudinally studied sample of physicians who participated in PHPs, psychiatrists were as likely as other physicians to be in practice after 5 years of treatment and monitoring. The philosophy and purpose of these programs are described at the Federation of State Physician Health Programs website (www.fsphp.org).

The American Psychological Association's ethical principles and code of conduct (available at www.apa.org/ethics/code/ethics-code-2017.pdf) are less specific than those of the American Medical Association (available at www.ama-assn.org/delivering-care/ethics/code-medical-ethics-overview)

TABLE 7–2.	Signs and symptoms of alcohol dependence that may appear in the workplace

Alcohol on the breath

Slurred speech

Unsteadiness

Tremor

Impaired memory and concentration

Erratic performance

Poor hygiene and dress

Lateness

Unexplained absences

Sweating

Irritability

Poor social behavior

Source. Adapted from Yellowlees P: *Physician Suicide: Cases and Commentaries.* Washington, DC, American Psychiatric Association Publishing, 2019, p. 117. Copyright © 2019 American Psychiatric Association. Used with permission.

and the American Psychiatric Association (available at www.psychiatry.org/psychiatrists/practice/ethics) regarding the issue of intervening with or reporting a colleague who may be impaired. State and provincial psychological associations are the best sources of additional information on programs available for colleagues.

Case Example 2

Kelly Greene is a division chief of a medium-sized academic department. A senior member of the department, Mary Keeney, now in her late 70s, is a valued and respected colleague, as well as a dedicated mentor to many junior faculty and trainees. Dr. Greene and Dr. Keeney have worked together for 15 years, and at one point, Dr. Keeney was Dr. Greene's supervisor when she was a resident. Over the last several years, Dr. Keeney has gradually started to show subtle, and not-so-subtle, signs of possible cognitive impairment. For example, during faculty meetings, she sometimes asks a question that is off topic or has already been discussed. The hospital has reported that Dr. Keeney has accumulated an increasing number of incomplete charts in the last year, and Dr. Greene is responsible for addressing this issue with her. She has missed several scheduled appointments with patients in the last several months, and when Dr. Greene asked her gently about it, she seemed flustered and became somewhat defensive, saying, "I have a lot on my plate!" In addition, Dr. Greene has noticed that Dr. Keeney has started to fall asleep during grand rounds, whereas she used to be an attentive and active participant.

Five years ago, Dr. Keeney suffered a fall while hiking with friends, sustained a concussion, and took 2 months' leave to recover. Initially, Dr. Greene and other faculty believe that the signs she is showing may be attributable to the residual effects of the concussion. Recently, however, a junior faculty member came to Dr. Greene and confidentially expressed concerns about Dr. Keeney's judgment in the care of several of her patients, as well as concerns that she was not responding to patients' messages. In addition, several patients have complained to the hospital's patient advocate in the last 6 months about Dr. Keeney's uncharacteristic behavior, including irritability toward patients. As Dr. Greene observes and hears about these signs of changes in performance, she begins to worry not only about Dr. Keeney's well-being and her patient care but also about the department's and institution's liability. Dr. Greene contemplates her ethical and legal obligations.

More than 29% of practicing physicians in the United States were age 60 or older in 2016, an increase from 25% in 2010. A greater proportion of male physicians (35.9%) than female physicians (15.7%) were 60 years or older in 2016. The aging of the physician workforce is increasingly on the radars of health systems, state medical boards, and professional societies (Kupfer 2016; LoboPrabhu et al. 2009). Although many psychiatrists and psychologists can continue to practice with high levels of competence late into life, aging is a risk factor for the development of cognitive impairment or neurocognitive disorders (NCDs), which include mild cognitive impairment or mild neurocognitive impairment, as well as dementias (major NCD) due to a variety of etiologies (e.g., Alzheimer's disease, vascular dementia, Lewy body disease, frontotemporal dementia, and other less frequent causes).

Screening, identification, and appropriate assessment and intervention with health professionals who may have (or may be developing) some form of NCD is an emerging area of research and policymaking. Although controversial, some health systems have implemented mandatory screening of their aging physicians for NCD. The behavior shown by Dr. Keeney demonstrates several potential warning signs of cognitive impairment (Table 7–3). If an individual shows changes in cognitive functioning such that compensatory strategies or accommodations are required to maintain independence or complete activities of daily living, a diagnosis of mild NCD may be applicable (American Psychiatric Association 2013).

TABLE 7–3. Signs and symptoms of cognitive impairment that may appear in the workplace

---

Impaired memory and concentration

Changes in documentation (e.g., sloppier work)

Absentmindedness (e.g., forgetting appointments)

Patient complaints

Changes in hygiene or dress

Lateness

Falling asleep

Apathy

Irritability

Changes in social behavior (e.g., inappropriate comments)

Dr. Keeney's lack of awareness of her condition is also typical; it is not at all uncommon for physicians with cognitive impairment to lack insight into their developing condition (Cooper et al. 2018). Because patient-clinician interactions often occur in private, with no one else present (this is particularly true in mental health professions), signs of cognitive impairment may go unnoticed and unreported for a long period of time (Cooper et al. 2018).

Of note, patient complaints may contain clues to physicians with NCD. Cooper et al. (2018) conducted a case-control study examining unsolicited patient complaints compiled in a large database (the Patient Advocacy Reporting System). They found that certain words distinguished physicians with a possible or probable NCD (*n* = 15) from two comparison groups of age- and sex-matched physicians (*n* = 60), matched by site and number of complaints. Physicians with NCD were 20 times more likely to have complaints that mentioned words suggestive of various domains of cognitive impairment (e.g., "forget," "confused," "inappropriate," "difficulty using"). The authors concluded that such words "reflect impairment domains [that] suggest the need for further testing rather than a definitive diagnosis" (Cooper et al. 2018, p. 935).

Individuals with mild NCD may still be able to function in their professional role, but—as in the case of substance use disorders—they may require careful assessment and monitoring. Additional restrictions on practice, as well as oversight, may be needed. Although there is currently no standard procedure for screening and management of health professionals with NCD, a variety of options are, nevertheless, available to concerned practitioners or colleagues. Because legal aspects of this area are evolving, it would be wise to seek out counsel from one's health care system (or its PHP) or professional society regarding the implications of referring (or not referring) a colleague to a PHP and of reporting (or not reporting) the colleague to the relevant licensing board.

Case Example 3

Art Garner is a 58-year-old physician on the faculty at a prestigious medical school. A conscientious clinician, beloved teacher, and highly valued colleague, Dr. Garner has had a fulfilling career and has been looking forward to stepping into a leadership role at the affiliated academic hospital in the coming year. His family has mentioned that it seems as if he is moving more slowly and speaking more deliberately, and his wife says that he looks as if he is gazing off into the distance. He has been having some difficulty sleeping and does not feel like running his usual 1- to 2-mile daily run because his back feels sore and his legs feel stiff. Dr. Garner says he feels "just the same" but notices that his conversations with patients, families, and colleagues do not have the same easy back-and-forth rhythm. He observes some awkwardness when speaking with medical students and residents. The time to complete his medical records has grown much longer. When his wife notices that he has an intermittent tremor, she asks him to go with her to see their physician. He is diagnosed with Parkinson's disease but is found to have no evidence of cognitive decline. He starts medication and has significant improvement in his symptoms. Soon thereafter, his division chief speaks with him about "problems at work," based on feedback from members of division and trainees, and a concern that he is not capable of assuming the new clinical leadership role.

Dr. Garner's situation raises a number of important considerations. His diagnosis of Parkinson's disease, although a risk factor, does not unequivocally imply impairment. The primary symptoms of this disorder include slower movements (bradykinesia) and tremor, both of which may be apparent to his colleagues. In addition, changes in mood are common. A patient may remain quite stable on medications for many years and, as in Dr. Garner's case, may not exhibit symptoms of cognitive impairment. The assumption in his case should be that he is capable of continuing to work but may need adaptations to his schedule, including longer times for clinical appointments and (if indicated) a reduced teaching or supervision load.

In this case, Dr. Garner has had a fairly comprehensive evaluation already, although the details of the neuropsychological assessment should be clarified. Although Dr. Garner is relatively young, some health care systems now require comprehensive evaluations for all practicing physicians older than a certain age (typically 70 or 75 years). For example, Stanford Hospital and Clinics adopted such a policy for the medical staff in 2012. Their Late Career Practitioner Policy applies to practitioners age 74.5 years or older who wish to obtain or maintain their clinical privileges. The initial policy required practitioners to undergo 1) peer assessment of their clinical performance, 2) a comprehensive history and physical (by a health care professional approved by the chair of the Credentials Committee, and 3) a cognitive screening conducted by an appointed evaluator. The cognitive screening component was removed in 2014 after concerns were raised by a group of older clinicians (Page 2015), many of whom felt they could continue to practice safely, sometimes with appropriate adaptations to their schedules or work assignments.

As the physician workforce continues to age, other health care systems will begin to implement similar policies. Examination of the processes and outcomes, as well as potential unintended consequences of such programs, will be critical to ensuring that they are deployed appropriately for the well-being of both clinicians and patients.

Case Example 4

Jason Stevens is a 56-year-old psychologist in private practice in a midsize city. Over the last 4 years, he has experienced multiple changes in his personal life. He and his wife had been growing apart for the last 10 years of their 30-year marriage, and when their two children left for college, their relationship declined to the point where his wife sought a divorce 2 years ago. She has since remarried and moved closer to one of their two children. Dr. Stevens, despite his outward appearance of functioning as before, has become increasingly sad, lonely, and depressed over the past year. He used to exercise 4–5 days a week but has stopped doing this in the past year. He feels he is under significant financial pressure due to the expenses of his children's education and doesn't feel he can afford to not see new patients or to take any time off from work to take care of himself. In addition, although he used to attend a monthly supervision group with five other psychologists, he stopped attending a year ago.

Six months ago, Dr. Stevens began treating a new psychotherapy patient, Shana, a single 33-year-old woman who is struggling with anxiety. Shana has a pattern of short-lived relationships with men while outwardly stating she wants to be in a committed relationship. As the psychotherapy progressed, Dr. Stevens found himself increasingly attracted to his patient. One month ago, at the end of a session, he hugged her after a particularly emotional discussion about her father. Over the last 3 weeks, each session has felt to him increasingly sexually charged. He has begun to ask Shana more specific questions than he had previously about her sexual encounters with men, justifying this to himself by saying that he simply wants to understand her better. In her most recent session with Dr. Stevens, in the context of lamenting her most recent breakup, Shana asks him directly if he has ever dated a patient. Feeling lonely and sensing that she is seducing him, Dr. Stevens winks at her and says, "Not yet, but what are you doing tonight?"

Is Dr. Stevens impaired? Although this scenario is different from the preceding ones in several ways (Dr. Stevens is not abusing substances and is not suffering from a physical disorder or an NCD), it nevertheless portrays a clinician who is showing signs of impaired judgment. Dr. Stevens has been increasingly crossing boundaries with his patient and unconsciously trying to meet his own emotional needs through her. He is particularly at risk given his recent life stressors, loneliness, and likely underlying psychological vulnerabilities. In addition, working in a private practice may put him at increased risk because he does not interact regularly with colleagues who might be able to support him.

Positive Practices

1. Learn the reporting requirement of the relevant jurisdiction (state or province) and licensing board.
2. Understand your obligations under your institution's code of conduct as well as your professional code of conduct.
3. Become aware of the different roles and responsibilities of licensing boards and PHPs.
4. Consider both patient safety and the well-being of yourself and your colleagues as an integral part of your professionalism and ethical obligation.
5. Realize that there are supports available for yourself and your colleagues and that these do not necessarily result in disciplinary or punitive actions by licensing boards.
6. Identify your institution's or organization's resources for reporting or inquiring about an impaired colleague. Physician wellness committees, ombudspersons, and other resources are in place at most organizations.
7. If you do become concerned about a colleague (or trainee or supervisor), the following options are all potentially useful, bearing in mind that different states have varying policies.

   - Consult with a trusted colleague about next steps.
   - Talk to your colleague about seeking help because being proactive is most likely to lead to positive (rather than punitive) outcomes.

- Consult with your health system's physician wellness committee.
- Consult with your local, regional, or state PHP about how to encourage your colleague to get help or how to refer your colleague.

Conclusion

Mental health professionals must be aware of the ethical and legal obligations to identify impairment. The well-being of psychiatrists and psychologists and that of their patients depends on a willingness to examine attitudes toward these issues as well as a willingness to confront them when they arise. Most mental health professionals will at some point in their careers encounter situations in which the competence of a colleague is subject to question. The issues related to discussing these concerns are complex and sensitive. It is important to remember that the presence of an illness does not in itself mean a colleague will experience impairment. A respectful approach to inquiring, providing support, and intervening only when necessary is critical.

Questions to Discuss With Colleagues and Mentors

—————o—————

- If I am concerned about one of my colleagues being impaired, what should I do? With whom can I talk confidentially?
- Whom do you call for advice when you are worried about a colleague?
- What resources exist in your workplace system for clinicians who are developing health, stress, and/or impairment issues?
- Have you yourself struggled with whether to refer a colleague for services?
- Have you had the experience of having to talk to a colleague about your concerns about his or her mental health or other issues, such as substance use?
- What kinds of issues come up when you do not refer a colleague for suspected health issues?

—————o—————

Recommended Resources

Gabbard GO: The role of compulsiveness in the normal physician. JAMA 254(20):2926–2929, 1985

Myers MF, Gabbard GO: The Physician as Patient: A Clinical Handbook
for Mental Health Professionals. Washington, DC, American Psychiatric Publishing, 2009

Wise EH, Hersh MA, Gibson CM: Ethics, self-care and well-being for
psychologists: reenvisioning the stress-distress continuum. Prof
Psychol Res Pract 43(5):487–494, 2012

Yellowlees PM, Campbell MD, Rose JS, et al: Psychiatrists with substance use disorders: positive treatment outcomes from physician
health programs. Psychiatr Serv 65(12):1492–1495, 2014

References

American Psychiatric Association: Diagnostic and Statistical Manual of Mental
Disorders, 5th Edition. Arlington, VA, American Psychiatric Association,
2013

Cooper WO, Martinez W, Domenico HJ, et al: Unsolicited patient complaints
identify physicians with evidence of neurocognitive disorders. Am J Geriatr
Psychiatry 26(9):927–936 2018

DesRoches CM, Rao SR, Fromson JA, et al: Physicians' perceptions, prepared-
ness for reporting, and experiences related to impaired and incompetent
colleagues. JAMA 304(2):187–193, 2010 20628132

Kupfer JM: The graying of US physicians: implications for quality and the future supply of physicians. JAMA 315(4):341–342, 2016 26720141

LoboPrabhu SM, Molinari VA, Hamilton JD, Lomax JW: The aging physician
with cognitive impairment: approaches to oversight, prevention, and remediation. Am J Geriatr Psychiatry 17(6):445–454, 2009 19461256

Page L: Should doctors be tested for competence at age 65? New York, Med-
scape, October 28, 2015. Available at: www.medscape.com/viewarticle/
848937_2. Accessed April 28, 2019.

Wynia MK: The role of professionalism and self-regulation in detecting impaired or incompetent physicians. JAMA 304(2):210–212, 2010 20628138

Yellowlees PM, Campbell MD, Rose JS, et al: Psychiatrists with substance use
disorders: positive treatment outcomes from physician health programs.
Psychiatr Serv 65(12):1492–1495, 2014 25270988

PART II

Well-Being and Positive Self-Care

Practical Approaches for Psychiatrists and Mental Health Professionals

ॐॐ

CHAPTER 8

Preventive Health Care Strategies: Fostering Positive Self-Care and Resilience

Resilience refers to the ability to adapt to a challenge, cope with a source of stress, or recover from an experience of adversity. The capacity to thrive in spite of life's many unpredictable struggles can be intentionally fostered. Psychiatrists and psychologists can take note of how much energy they expend and can conserve their energy by avoiding tasks that are too draining. Mental health clinicians can also determine the behaviors that help them to recharge or regain energy so that they can remain strong for new challenges. Access to greater physical, mental, and emotional resources can allow psychiatrists or psychologists to remain calm, think clearly, and avoid becoming overwhelmed even in stressful situations.

Part II of this book focuses on practical steps that mental health clinicians can take to better care for themselves and to promote their own resilience. The goal of Part II is much greater than simply preventing burnout and negative outcomes; the goal is to support psychiatrists and psychologists in living healthy and fulfilling lives with meaningful personal connections and professional contributions.

The individual is the most powerful force in promoting his or her own well-being. In this chapter and the following chapters, we focus on specific life domains that have a major impact on well-being, including physical activity, diet, sleep, social connection, therapy and psychiatric care, spirituality and mindfulness, and meaningful work. No one is alone on the journey to self-care and resilience; struggles in some or all of these life domains are a central part of what it means to be human. Seeking a meaningful, connected, and healthy life is the first step to promoting well-being.

In the spirit of mindfulness and self-compassion, readers need to be kind to themselves. In Part II, we provide resources and ideas for self-care, but readers should not overburden themselves with lengthy to-do lists. Try self-gratitude when reading about a strategy you already employ and appreciate the impact of this strategy on your resilience or well-being. When reading about an area of life in need of attention, take a mindful approach. Pay attention to which of the proposed strategies is most naturally appealing. Work on nonjudgmental awareness regarding the possibility of pursuing new actions to further support well-being. Try not to take blame for what has not yet been done. Be patient with the process.

Benefits: The Case for Positive Self-Care and Resilience Practices

Psychiatrists and psychologists know a great deal about promoting resilience, whether through therapy approaches, relaxation techniques, or the process of changing daily habits. Mental health clinicians also have great psychological resources to draw on to support their own mental health. What would one tell a patient struggling to change a habit, coping with a challenging life experience, or managing persistent negative emotions? What tools are most effective for individuals in treatment? Many of the treatment strategies for promoting mood stabilization, reducing anxiety, building healthy interpersonal relationships, or promoting healthy eating or sleep patterns are highly applicable to self-care. Individuals can use what they already know.

A rapidly growing body of evidence supports the strong role of self-care in enhancing physical health, energy, mood, mental well-being, and resilience in the face of challenging life circumstances. The positive psychology movement (Seligman and Csikszentmihalyi 2000; Seligman et al. 2005) has already had significant influence on the field of psychiatry and mental health care. Some researchers refer to the concept of *flourishing*, an optimal state of resilience in which an individual is able to grow personally and can help others do the same (Moutier 2013). Figure 8–1 outlines the continuum of well-being for professionals.

Negative outcomes are not the inevitable consequence of stressful experiences; great fulfillment can be found through the cultivation of one's capacity for resilience (Schaufeli et al. 2009; Seligman et al. 2005; Wise et al. 2012). The intentional application of positive wellness prac-

Negative factors	Positive factors
Poor health	Good health
Lack of purpose	Strong sense of purpose
Excessive stress	Stimulation and engagement
Poor coping style	Adaptive coping style
Poor mentorship and supervision	Mentorship and supervision
Inadequate psychosocial support	Strong psychosocial support
Interpersonal conflict	Harmonious relationships
Excessive work demands	Appropriate work demands
Adverse work environment	Constructive work environment

The well-being continuum

Languishing - Flourishing

FIGURE 8–1. The well-being continuum.

Factors influencing the well-being of professionals.
Source. Copyright © 2015 Laura Weiss Roberts, M.D., M.A.

tices can have surprisingly beneficial effects, even among individuals who have experienced great trauma or adversity (Lyubomirsky et al. 2005; Seligman et al. 2005). Physicians who deliberately cultivate their own wellness have been found to have higher levels of overall well-being (Irving et al. 2009; Weiner et al. 2001). Psychologists who cultivate balance between their personal and professional lives, maintain meaningful relationships outside of work, take vacations, and engage in therapy have been found to have enhanced psychological well-being as well (Coster and Schwebel 1997).

The science of clinician well-being is now considered a legitimate field, drawing insights and potential solutions from psychiatry, psychology, sports medicine, nutrition, spiritual care, education, law, and economics. There is hope that the well-being movement can inspire future generations of psychiatrists and psychologists to attend to their own self-care, which will, in turn, benefit society at large. The positive impact that one can and will have on the world depends directly on one's own well-being and resilience.

Barriers to Self-Care

Serious barriers can stand in the way of achieving better self-care. Evidence suggests that certain medical specialties, including psychiatry, may experience particularly high emotional burden as part of their routine practice (Seritan 2013). The work of any psychiatrist or psychologist can be emotionally draining because of the near-constant exposure to human suffering. Additionally, the current health care system emphasizes quantity over quality, which may encourage unrealistic self-sacrifice on the part of health care workers. When clinicians are under pressure, they may work even harder, but professional satisfaction and productivity are not increased for those who work longer hours (Balch et al. 2010). In fact, working longer hours may increase the risk of medical errors, contribute to burnout, and even erode personal relationships that could otherwise serve as protective factors in stressful circumstances (Seritan 2013).

Trainees may face specific barriers to self-care. Lack of control over work schedules and job expectations has been found to be a significant stressor (Scheurer et al. 2009; Shanafelt et al. 2009). Although this is a serious problem for staff and faculty, trainees often function in systems where they have little authority and even less control. Furthermore, trainees may become emotionally vulnerable when they first encounter serious mental illness or instances of abuse. First exposure to trauma, for instance, has been associated with greater risk of vicarious traumatization.

Overcoming Barriers to Self-Care

Evidence suggests that physicians are not very good at accurately judging how well they are engaging in self-care (Shanafelt and Noseworthy 2017). At the organizational level, psychiatrists and psychologists can periodically assess variables related to clinician well-being and can calibrate their impressions on the basis of feedback and benchmarking information. Evidence suggests that providing objective information to clinicians about how their well-being compares with other similar clinicians on a national scale can help inspire a change in behavior (Shanafelt et al. 2014).

Organizations can also make the importance of self-care explicit by offering resources to support clinician well-being (e.g., clear policies related to time off, benefits for dependent care, healthy food choices on site, access to employee assistance programs for medical and mental health care). Direct training for clinicians to promote personal resilience can also have beneficial effects. Evidence suggests that even brief interventions to promote resilience can have significant effects. For instance, in their wait-list controlled study, Sood and colleagues (2011) investigated the effects of Stress Management and Resilience Training (SMART), which focused on 1) attention to the present moment and to the novelty of the world and 2) flexible rather than fixed interpretation of experiences and deliberate cultivation of gratitude, compassion, and acceptance. Compared with the control group, faculty physicians participating in the SMART intervention reported feeling greater resilience and quality of life, with lower perceived stress and anxiety after a single 90-minute session.

Whether motivated to improve one's own health or attempting to improve the self-care of trainees or employees on an organizational level, a clear understanding of the dynamics that support and detract from self-care can help guide decision-making about where to invest the most energy. It may also be helpful to reflect on the types of change strategies that have been useful in the past, either for oneself or for those being helped. For some people, understanding the science and the rationale behind a recommended practice helps motivate change. For others, it is more important to solve practical issues and put structural supports in place for accountability. Approach the process like a scientist; try out ideas and gather data to see if a hypothesis is supported. Find small changes supported by your own data that make a big difference in wellness.

One helpful data-gathering technique is to track how time is spent over the course of a week (e.g., creating a daily grid with hourly entries, Table 8–1). Often, just by writing down a simple time log, you can gain insight into your patterns and an understanding about what needs to change. Complete the log from memory, looking back over the past week, or use a log in the coming week to capture how time is actually spent. Some people even find a time log to be helpful for future planning, filling out when they assume future plans will be completed and then checking the accuracy of those assumptions later.

Once the log is complete, notice whether any activities occur with surprising frequency. Also, try to notice what might be missing from the week. Keep these impressions in mind while reading the rest of the chapter, and then complete the exercises at the end of the chapter.

Change and Flexibility Across the Professional Life Span

Self-care strategies that are effective during one stage of a person's life may need to be significantly altered to accommodate changing personal or professional roles and responsibilities. For instance, many professionals find that they must either tailor the strategies they used during training or seek out new strategies to fit their lives as part of the professional workforce. Significant life events may disrupt healthy habits;

TABLE 8–1.   Weekly time log

	Mon.	Tues.	Wed.	Thurs.	Fri.	Sat.	Sun.
5A.M.							
6A.M.							
7A.M.							
8A.M.							
9A.M.							
10A.M.							
11A.M.							
12P.M.							
1P.M.							
2P.M.							
3P.M.							
4P.M.							
5P.M.							
6P.M.							
7P.M.							
8P.M.							
9P.M.							
10P.M.							
11P.M.							

when a clinician becomes a parent or takes responsibility for caring for an aging family member, new self-care strategies may be needed. The following two vignettes provide positive examples of how professionals sometimes deal with these challenges.

Vignette

Julie Kitahama, a family therapist, found that finding time to exercise was much more difficult once she had young children at home. She realized that between inconsistent sleep and her efforts to be productive at work, she was not getting any regular exercise. She decided to seek advice from a more senior colleague. The colleague disclosed that she was experiencing the same problem because her husband had recently undergone hip replacement surgery and no longer could join her for daily walks. She and her colleague decided to use their lunch break at work to fit in a bit of exercise, going for a walk or a run. By taking a slightly longer lunch, they were able to sign up for and attend a swim class together 1 or 2 days per week. Other colleagues were inspired by these visible efforts, and the motivation to exercise spread across their department. Exercise became a valuable way to expand professional connections and increase morale. Explicit acknowledgment of the benefits of exercise helped motivate others to create small exercise groups based on individual interests. Looking back several years later, Ms. Kitahama realized that making the personal commitment to find time during the workday to exercise inspired her to be more productive when she was working.

Vignette

Gustav Monroe was a social worker in a community-based mental health clinic serving teens with history of trauma for 15 years when his brother was diagnosed with an aggressive brain tumor. He decided to take a leave of absence to better support his brother and cope with his own grief and loss. When he was ready to return to work at the clinic, he met with his supervisor to discuss the types of cases he wanted to take on going forward. He found that he was now greatly interested in helping young children undergoing cancer treatment. Although his recent personal experience with his brother made pursuing this interest emotionally difficult, he decided to enroll in additional training to develop expertise in helping children with life-threatening medical illnesses. With support from his clinical management team, he arranged his schedule to accommodate an evening class. He also started attending grand rounds at the local hospital to learn more about current research in pediatric oncology. Eventually, he decided to apply for a job in the consultation-liaison service. In his new role, he felt that he was able to make a difference for children and families struggling with some of the same issues his brother had faced. Although Mr. Monroe maintained an interest in work with childhood trauma, the emphasis on pediatric oncology brought greater meaning to his life.

Components of Resilience

Resilience and positive self-care are fundamental aspects of healthy living, and when they are compromised, they can be significant contributors to professional burnout and many other health complications (Roberts and Trockel 2019). Many of these strategies are "fuel" for achieving the life one desires (Dunn et al. 2008). Self-care activities might also be seen as "recharging" one's internal battery and contributing to resilience (Figure 8–2). While some experiences, such as chronic

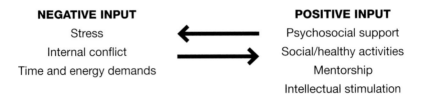

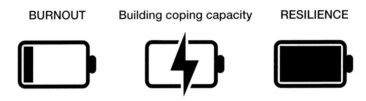

FIGURE 8–2. Recharging one's batteries for resilience.

Source. Adapted from Dunn et al. 2008.

sleep deprivation, are draining and contribute to burnout, others, such as receiving social support, are restorative and contribute to resilience. When one frequently seeks out restorative activities, one will have enough energy to cope with challenges without completely depleting energy stores.

Physical Health

The first aspect of positive self-care relates to physical needs. Physical needs include exercise, nutrition, and sleep, as well as routine medical care. The busy lifestyle of a modern-day professional can make it difficult to take care of one's body. Evidence suggests that at least half of U.S. adults have at least one chronic illness (National Center for Chronic Disease Prevention and Health Promotion 2019), making care for the physical body even more important. Although psychiatrists and psychologists may sacrifice sleep or physical activity to meet work and family demands, compromised physical health undermines performance in all areas.

With a growing body of literature supporting the many positive and preventive health benefits of physical exercise, the World Health Organization (2018) has called for greater emphasis on physical activity in health care across the life span. The clear connection between sedentary behavior and many chronic diseases (Thompson et al. 2003) highlights the importance of this recommendation for prevention and management of a diverse range of chronic conditions, including heart disease, cancer, diabetes, and mental illness (Blair 2009; O'Donoghue et al. 2011). Regular exercise also provides mental health benefits. Healthy body composition has been linked to multiple aspects of psychological well-being, such as greater self-esteem and lower stress (Guest and Smith-Coggins 2013).

Diet has tremendous effects on energy, mood, and longevity and is significantly influenced by environmental conditions, including workplace stress. In a Chinese study published in the *Journal of Applied Psychology*, Liu and colleagues (2017) reported the relationship between job demands and food consumption in 125 information technology workers. Results indicated that the experience of high job demands had a negative effect on healthy eating patterns later the same day. In another study, employees with healthier eating habits were 25% more likely to report high job performance ratings compared with employees who reported unhealthy eating habits (Merrill et al. 2013).

Sleep and adequate rest are the body's most basic way of regaining energy. An explosion of sleep research over the past several decades has affirmed the central role that sleep plays in energy, productivity, and mental health. Unusual sleep patterns (both chronic lack of sleep and excessive sleep) have been associated with greater mortality (Ferrie et al. 2007; Tamakoshi et al. 2004). Lack of sleep has been linked to greater risk of heart disease (Ayas et al. 2003; Liu et al. 2002), inflammation (Irwin et al. 2010), and cognitive impairments (Alhola and Polo-Kantola 2007; Van Dongen et al. 2003). Many psychiatrists and psychologists find, however, that they need to catch up on documentation or other scholarly tasks during the evening hours. Ironically, this time would be better invested in improving efficiencies of practice. With inadequate sleep, productivity is poor and rates of errors skyrocket. Even more concerning is the fact that sleep-deprived individuals may think they are functioning well even when they are actually impaired (Harrison and Horne 2000).

Social Relationships

Positive self-care must involve the cultivation of strong social relationships. Whether focusing on cultivating a feeling of community in the workplace or carving out quality time with friends and family, having a strong social connection with others is beneficial. In one of the most comprehensive longitudinal studies to date, now running for more than 80 years, researchers from the Harvard Study of Adult Development (www.adultdevelopmentstudy.org) repeatedly found that happiness is associated with relationship satisfaction and social connections across the life span (Waldinger and Schulz 2010).

Relationship quality has surprisingly strong effects on physical and mental health, and these effects can be either positive or negative. Increased risk for conditions such as heart disease, cancer, addiction, and depression in those who lack social connections has been reported. For instance, people who are in committed romantic relationships have been found to have lower risk of heart disease (Smith and Baucom 2017). Strong social relationships also increase an individual's survival odds by up to 50%, according to a meta-analysis of 148 studies (Holt-Lunstad et al. 2010).

Social connection influences health through many pathways. Biologically, social connection influences such factors as immune function and stress hormones (Uchino and Way 2017). Behaviorally, social connection influences health-related habits. For instance, research suggests that relationship intimacy is associated with lower levels of cortisol (Ditzen et al. 2008). In addition, people in supportive relationships may be more likely to engage in lifestyle behaviors, often with others, that support their long-term health.

Many people find great fulfillment from connecting with people who share their interests. Professionals might join a book club or schedule periodic outings with colleagues, which may enhance both personal and professional feelings of support. An additional advantage of finding colleagues who share one's personal interests is that these colleagues can enhance one's sense of connectedness and community at work. Interest groups can be formed around areas of professional interest at work, whether for the purpose of case consultation or for scholarly pursuits, such as a writing group.

In the workplace, a sense of community and connections with colleagues have been found to reduce burnout (Shanafelt et al. 2017; Van Ham et al. 2006). Similarly, connection with others in general is known to be an important protective factor against isolation and burnout (Jibson 2013). Still, little scientific work has focused on factors to enhance morale in the workplace. The best practice is likely to cultivate multiple sources of support. Meaningful connection with colleagues can be found during collaboration on a project of mutual interest. Department social activities can improve efficiency as well as boost morale. Regional and professional associations can also be an important source of professional support and practical information.

Time with friends and family members outside of the workplace can also yield essential support. Some professionals may also want to formalize a therapy or executive coaching relationship to further support their growth and development. Given how many people find that they thrive from social connection, no matter the specific approach, strengthening professional and personal relationships is likely to have an effect on well-being (Moutier 2013).

Mental and Emotional Well-Being

Emotional health is another critical aspect of self-care. Studies even suggest that emotional well-being is tied to multiple physical health metrics (Ryff et al. 2006). Individuals may be rewarded with powerful benefits from training to enhance emotional well-being or pursuing emotional well-being interventions. Greater attention to emotional health may take many forms, whether involving formal psychotherapy, religious activity, a mindfulness practice, or a relationship with emotionally supportive family or colleagues (Irving et al. 2009). Strategies such as stress inoculation, relaxation, and meditation may be beneficial in some cases. Training related to time management, assertiveness, or other interpersonal social skills may also be useful (Maslach et al. 2001). Positive reframing has been suggested as a tool many practitioners may be able to employ. Positive reframing involves asking questions designed to broaden a person's mental perspective, such as "How would another person handle this situation?" "Will this matter to me in 6 months or a year?" and "Is there a chance to learn something useful from this?" (Schwartz 2007; Seritan 2013). Incorporating gratitude and compassion into one's philosophy may be particularly beneficial.

Practices supporting emotional and mental health can be incorporated into the workplace. In fact, maintaining mental and emotional health is considered a core aspect of professionalism and ethical practice (Shanafelt et al. 2017). Research has suggested that mindfulness can be embedded into corporate culture, with beneficial effects on employee stress management, teamwork, and focus (Good et al. 2016). Effective physician-patient communication has been consistently associated with better patient outcomes (Stewart 1995), and preliminary evidence indicates that therapist mindfulness training is also associated with patient symptom improvement (Grepmair et al. 2007). Addressing physician burnout by offering resources related to work-life integration, resilience, and positive psychology has also been suggested (Back et al. 2016; Epstein 1999; Krasner et al. 2009; Novack et al. 1997). By attending to their emotional health, psychiatrists and psychologists will benefit from improved mental focus, flexibility, and ability to incorporate multiple points of view.

Meaningful Professional Contribution

Finding meaning in one's work is a strong predictor of professional satisfaction and personal well-being. Feelings of limited control and lack of impact may lead to burnout. Feeling active and effective and being recognized for one's accomplishments at work lead to engagement. Inevitable fatigue and frustration are much easier to handle when work is perceived as meaningful. Even the very real challenges of mental health care can be mitigated by the sense that work is making a difference for good.

A sense of meaning in work is highly individual. Some health care professionals may find clinical care to be the most meaningful. Other professionals may value research or teaching. Others may consider leadership, administration, or policy work to be most important. The key is to understand oneself and, above all, find a way to follow one's passions, whatever they may be. Evidence suggests that spending even the equivalent of 1 day per week on an activity of personal meaning has substantial benefits for professional satisfaction (Shanafelt et al. 2009).

Most professionals find that working with others enhances their sense of purpose at work. It is rare that a professional will be able to complete a meaningful project without substantial collaboration from others. Providing mentorship and helping the next generation of trainees can also make work feel purposeful. Opportunities to acknowledge colleagues for meaningful contributions and to reflect on remarkable work done by others can be highly beneficial for both organizational morale and personal long-term resilience.

Financial Health

Financial strain can also negatively affect practitioner well-being. The first step to financial health is to be informed about financial issues likely to affect career and family life. Unfortunately, professional training does not involve much financial education, and it can be difficult to find sound advice about personal finances or training in how to manage professional financial decisions.

Many mental health professionals begin their careers with substantial debt from college, medical school, or graduate education. This type of debt can complicate decision-making about the type of job to pursue after completing school. Getting out of debt requires particularly focused and consistent effort over many years. Although some professionals may take advantage of loan repayment programs, allowing for some debt forgiveness in exchange for services, other professionals need to make steady progress to reduce debt on their own.

As professionals advance in their careers, both personal and professional finances typically become more complex. Although earning potential often grows with experience, personal expenses may also expand as an individual balances care for family members in the short term with longer-term expenditures (e.g., mortgage, children's college tuition, retirement). For instance, when a health professional returns to work after maternity or paternity leave, the cost of childcare can be substantial. Decisions about how much to work and what types of work to pursue have major implications for both financial health and other aspects of personal wellness. In addition, learning the ins and outs of budgeting and financial planning for clinical programs is often necessary. Like other aspects of well-being, this is a place where good mentorship will make a big difference. Determine what knowledge is needed and look for colleagues who can offer advice and guidance.

Another important aspect of financial health relates to making sure spending aligns with values. The best practice is likely different for each individual. After reflecting on personal values, make a plan to spend money only on things that make a real difference. Keep in mind that some purchases have a disproportionate effect on happiness. For instance, across samples of adults in the United States, Denmark, Canada, and the Netherlands, data indicate that people who paid others to do tasks, such as housework, shopping, and cooking, rated their life satisfaction higher than those who spent money in other ways. In the lives of busy professionals, using money to save time appears to bring more positive benefits than material purchases do (Whillans et al. 2017).

Do What You Know, But for Yourself

Think about the types of self-care strategies that you typically recommend when providing counseling or psychotherapy to patients. Perhaps you often counsel patients to attend to sleep hygiene, get more regular exercise, or schedule special time with a child or partner. Professionals can apply to themselves the skills they know and teach, such as active coping strategies, reframing, and mindfulness. Telling a patient that it is important to take vacations or visit a primary health professional regularly might be easy, but this sound advice is easier to give than to follow.

Do an honest self-check about whether benefit can be gained from focusing personally on these strategies.

Positive Practices

1. Take a few minutes now to reflect on your own self-care in each of the domains discussed in this chapter. Consider whether there are any areas where you do particularly well taking care of yourself. Are there areas you already know you need to give more attention?

   - How well are you taking care of your physical health? Do you manage to get exercise on a regular basis? Do you get adequate sleep? Eat nutritious meals? Visit the doctor regularly?
   - Do you get at least some quality time with your children or partner each week? Do you have regular opportunities for connection with friends and extended family members? Do you have meaningful personal connections with colleagues at work?
   - What are you doing to nurture your emotional and mental health? For example, do you maintain a sense of mindfulness or gratitude, talk with a therapist, or participate in religious activities?
   - At work, are you able to spend at least some time each week on a project that is personally meaningful to you?
   - How is your financial health? Do you have a plan for paying off any debts from training? Are you saving for retirement or another important financial goal?

2. This coming week, try the following experiment: At least once each day, work briefly on the project of highest importance to you, before you do anything else. Pay attention to how this makes you feel. Many professionals find that consistent work on a meaningful project improves their overall sense of well-being. Consider whether you can commit to working on your most meaningful project at least 15 minutes each day or at least an hour each week.

3. Consider the tasks that you do on a regular basis that you find burdensome. Can you invest financial resources to get more help with one of those tasks?

4. Many people find that their own sense of well-being is vastly improved when they do small acts to help others. Take a moment to think about someone you know who is struggling with a stressful life event or personal circumstance. Maybe you have a colleague who is just returning to work after the birth of a child or a loved one's serious illness. Maybe you can think of someone suddenly doing extra

work because a colleague left the organization. Maybe you know someone who just moved to the area and might need someone to show him or her around. Offer to help this friend or colleague and take note of how it feels to help someone in need.

Conclusion

This chapter is the introduction to Part II of the book, which focuses on practical steps that psychiatrists and psychologists can take to better care for themselves and to promote their own resilience. The goal of Part II is to support psychiatrists and psychologists in living healthy and fulfilling lives with meaningful personal connections and professional contributions. In subsequent chapters, we provide more detail on each topic. While reading these chapters, take a mindful approach to self-evaluation. Remember that these are lifelong processes that all professionals go through in order to grow and develop. One must embrace compassion for oneself while making changes in one's life.

Exercises

The following are additional ideas for practical steps to take when enhancing resilience.

1. **Schedule your "must-haves."** Write down essential things that *must* be part of your life, such as sleep, exercise, and connection with loved ones. Take a moment to add these to your calendar to help keep them from getting overlooked as you get busy.

   _____

   _____

   _____

2. **Experiment with energy management.** Spend a few days paying attention to the types of activities that seem to give you energy and the types of activities that drain your energy. These are different for each person, but once you know what they are, you can deliberately adjust the order or amount of particular activities to achieve more balance. For instance,

make sure there are not just energy-expending activities but also energizing activities (sleep, nutrition, or work on a ful-filling project) sprinkled throughout the day or week to make life seem more balanced.

Write down three tasks or activities that reliably drain your energy.

_____

_____

_____

Write down three tasks or activities that usually make you feel inspired or eager to act.

_____

_____

_____

When you know you will be doing a draining activity, how could you plan to add an energizing task as well?

_____

_____

_____

3. **Practice gratitude.** List three good things that happen each day. These can be personal or professional and can be something you did or just something you noticed.

_____

_____

_____

Take a moment to look over this list and send a mental message of gratitude.

4. **Self-reflect.** As you read this chapter, you may have had some thoughts about aspects of your personal well-being that need improvement. First, write down a few things you are doing well.

_____

_____

_____

Now, make a list of at least three areas of wellness that are under your control and you wish to improve.

_____

_____

_____

5. **Pick a priority.** Take a moment to look over the list above, and select one of the items you would like to prioritize. Consider an initial step you may want to take to enhance this aspect of well-being.

_____

_____

_____

———————O———————

Recommended Resources

Brach T: Radical Acceptance: Embracing Your Life With the Heart of a Buddha. New York, Bantam, 2004

Dunn LB, Iglewicz A, Moutier C: A conceptual model of medical student well-being: promoting resilience and preventing burnout. Acad Psychiatry 32(1):44–53, 2008

Moutier C: How to have a healthy life balance as an academic physician, in The Academic Medicine Handbook: A Guide to Achievement and Fulfillment for Academic Faculty. Edited by Roberts LW, New York, Springer, 2013, pp 429–435

Noordsy DL (ed): Lifestyle Psychiatry. Washington, DC, American Psychiatric Association Publishing, 2019

Palmer BW (ed): Positive Psychiatry: A Clinical Handbook. Arlington, VA, American Psychiatric Association Publishing, 2015

PRI/PRX and the Greater Good Science Center: The science of happiness (podcast). Berkeley, CA, Greater Good Science Center, launched 2018. Available at: https://greatergood.berkeley.edu/podcasts and https://podcasts.apple.com/us/podcast/the-science-of-happiness/id1340505607. Accessed January 2, 2020.

Rath T: Eat Move Sleep: How Small Choices Lead to Big Changes. Arlington, VA, Missionday, 2013

Seritan AL: How to recognize and avoid burnout, in The Academic Medicine Handbook: A Guide to Achievement and Fulfillment for Academic Faculty. Edited by Roberts LW. New York, Springer, 2013, pp 447–453

Summers RF, Jeste DV: Positive Psychiatry: A Casebook. Washington, DC, American Psychiatric Association Publishing, 2019

Vanderkam L: What the Most Successful People Do Before Breakfast and Two Other Short Guides to Achieving More at Work and at Home. New York, Penguin, 2013

References

Alhola P, Polo-Kantola P: Sleep deprivation: impact on cognitive performance. Neuropsychiatr Dis Treat 3(5):553–567, 2007 19300585

Ayas NT, White DP, Manson JE, et al: A prospective study of sleep duration and coronary heart disease in women. Arch Intern Med 163(2):205–209, 2003 12546611

Back AL, Steinhauser KE, Kamal AH, Jackson VA: Building resilience for palliative care clinicians: an approach to burnout prevention based on individual skills and workplace factors. J Pain Symptom Manage 52(2):284–291, 2016 26921494

Balch CM, Shanafelt TD, Dyrbye L, et al: Surgeon distress as calibrated by hours worked and nights on call. J Am Coll Surg 211(5):609–619, 2010 20851643

Blair SN: Physical inactivity: the biggest public health problem of the 21st century. Br J Sports Med 43(1):1–2, 2009 19136507

Coster JS, Schwebel M: Well-functioning in professional psychologists. Prof Psychol Res Pr 28(1):5–13, 1997

Ditzen B, Hoppmann C, Klumb P: Positive couple interactions and daily cortisol: on the stress-protecting role of intimacy. Psychosom Med 70(8):883–889, 2008 18842747

Dunn LB, Iglewicz A, Moutier C: A conceptual model of medical student well-being: promoting resilience and preventing burnout. Acad Psychiatry 32(1):44–53, 2008 18270280

Epstein RM: Mindful practice. JAMA 282(9):833–839, 1999 10478689

Ferrie JE, Shipley MJ, Cappuccio FP, et al: A prospective study of change in sleep duration: associations with mortality in the Whitehall II cohort. Sleep 30(12):1659–1666, 2007 18246975

Good DJ, Lyddy CJ, Glomb TM, et al: Contemplating mindfulness at work: an integrative review. J Manage 42(1):114–142, 2016

Grepmair L, Mitterlehner F, Loew T, et al: Promoting mindfulness in psychotherapists in training influences the treatment results of their patients: a randomized, double-blind, controlled study. Psychother Psychosom 76(6):332–338, 2007 17917468

Guest C, Smith-Coggins R: How to care for the basics: sleep, nutrition, exercise, health, in The Academic Medicine Handbook: A Guide to Achievement and Fulfillment for Academic Faculty. Edited by Roberts LW. New York, Springer, 2013, pp 437–445

Harrison Y, Horne JA: The impact of sleep deprivation on decision making: a review. J Exp Psychol Appl 6(3):236–249, 2000, 11014055

Holt-Lunstad J, Smith TB, Layton JB: Social relationships and mortality risk: a meta-analytic review. PLoS Med 7(7):e1000316, 2010 20668659

Irving JA, Dobkin PL, Park J: Cultivating mindfulness in health care professionals: a review of empirical studies of mindfulness-based stress reduction (MBSR). Complement Ther Clin Pract 15(2):61–66, 2009 19341981

Irwin MR, Carrillo C, Olmstead R: Sleep loss activates cellular markers of inflammation: sex differences. Brain Behav Immun 24(1):54–57, 2010 19520155

Jibson MD: How to strengthen your own and others' morale, in The Academic Medicine Handbook: A Guide to Achievement and Fulfillment for Academic Faculty. Edited by Roberts LW. New York, Springer, 2013, pp 343–354

Krasner MS, Epstein RM, Beckman H, et al: Association of an educational program in mindful communication with burnout, empathy, and attitudes among primary care physicians. JAMA 302(12):1284–1293, 2009 19773563

Liu Y, Tanaka H, Fukuoka Heart Study Group: Overtime work, insufficient sleep, and risk of non-fatal acute myocardial infarction in Japanese men. Occup Environ Med 59(7):447–451, 2002 12107292

Liu Y, Song Y, Koopmann J, et al: Eating your feelings? Testing a model of employees' work-related stressors, sleep quality, and unhealthy eating. J Appl Psychol 102(8):1237–1258, 2017 28394149

Lyubomirsky S, Sheldon KM, Schkade D: Pursuing happiness: the architecture of sustainable change. Rev Gen Psychol 9(2):111–131, 2005

Maslach C, Schaufeli WB, Leiter MP: Job burnout. Annu Rev Psychol 52:397–422, 2001 11148311

Merrill RM, Aldana SG, Pope JE, et al: Self-rated job performance and absenteeism according to employee engagement, health behaviors, and physical health. J Occup Environ Med 55(1):10–18, 2013 23254387

Moutier C: How to have a healthy life balance as an academic physician, in The Academic Medicine Handbook: A Guide to Achievement and Fulfillment for Academic Faculty. Edited by Roberts LW. New York, Springer, 2013, pp 429–435

National Center for Chronic Disease Prevention and Health Promotion: About Chronic Diseases. Atlanta, GA, Centers for Disease Control and Prevention, 2019. Available at: www.cdc.gov/chronicdisease/about/index.htm. Accessed July 2019.

Novack DH, Suchman AL, Clark W, et al: Calibrating the physician: personal awareness and effective patient care. Working Group on Promoting Physician Personal Awareness, American Academy on Physician and Patient. JAMA 278(6):502–509, 1997 9256226

O'Donoghue G, Doody C, Cusack T: Physical activity and exercise promotion and prescription in undergraduate physiotherapy education: content analysis of Irish curricula. Physiotherapy 97(2):145–153, 2011 21497249

Roberts LW, Trockel MT (eds): The Art and Science of Physician Wellbeing: A Handbook for Physicians and Trainees. Cham, Switzerland, Springer, 2019

Ryff CD, Dienberg Love G, Urry HL, et al: Psychological well-being and ill-being: do they have distinct or mirrored biological correlates? Psychother Psychosom 75(2):85–95, 2006 16508343

Schaufeli WB, Leiter MP, Maslach C: Burnout: 35 years of research and practice. Career Development International 14(3):204–220, 2009

Scheurer D, McKean S, Miller J, Wetterneck T: U.S. physician satisfaction: a systematic review. J Hosp Med 4(9):560–568, 2009 20013859

Schwartz T: Manage your energy, not your time. Harv Bus Rev 85(10):63–164, 2007 17972496

Seligman MEP, Csikszentmihalyi M: Positive psychology: an introduction. Am Psychol 55(1):5–14, 2000 11392865

Seligman MEP, Steen TA, Park N, Peterson C: Positive psychology progress: empirical validation of interventions. Am Psychol 60(5):410–421, 2005 16045394

Seritan AL: How to recognize and avoid burnout, in The Academic Medicine Handbook: A Guide to Achievement and Fulfillment for Academic Faculty. Edited by Roberts LW. New York, Springer, 2013, pp 447–453

Shanafelt TD, Noseworthy JH: Executive leadership and physician well-being: nine organizational strategies to promote engagement and reduce burnout. Mayo Clin Proc 92(1):129–146, 2017 27871627

Shanafelt TD, West CP, Sloan JA, et al: Career fit and burnout among academic faculty. Arch Intern Med 169(10):990–995, 2009 19468093

Shanafelt TD, Kaups KL, Nelson H, et al: An interactive individualized intervention to promote behavioral change to increase personal well-being in US surgeons. Ann Surg 259(1):82–88, 2014 23979287

Shanafelt TD, Dyrbye LN, West CP: Addressing physician burnout: the way forward. JAMA 317(9):901–902, 2017 28196201

Smith TW, Baucom BRW: Intimate relationships, individual adjustment, and coronary heart disease: implications of overlapping associations in psychosocial risk. Am Psychol 72(6):578–589, 2017 28880104

Sood A, Prasad K, Schroeder D, Varkey P: Stress management and resilience training among Department of Medicine faculty: a pilot randomized clinical trial. J Gen Intern Med 26(8):858–861, 2011 21279454

Stewart MA: Effective physician-patient communication and health outcomes: a review. CMAJ 152(9):1423–1433, 1995 7728691

Tamakoshi A, Ohno Y, JACC Study Group: Self-reported sleep duration as a predictor of all-cause mortality: results from the JACC study, Japan. Sleep 27(1):51–54, 2004 14998237

Thompson PD, Buchner D, Piña IL, et al: Exercise and physical activity in the prevention and treatment of atherosclerotic cardiovascular disease: a statement from the Council on Clinical Cardiology (Subcommittee on Exercise, Rehabilitation, and Prevention) and the Council on Nutrition, Physical Activity, and Metabolism (Subcommittee on Physical Activity). Circulation 107(24):3109–3116, 2003 12821592

Uchino BN, Way BM: Integrative pathways linking close family ties to health: a neurochemical perspective. Am Psychol 72(6):590–600, 2017 28880105

Van Dongen HPA, Maislin G, Mullington JM, Dinges DF: The cumulative cost of additional wakefulness: dose-response effects on neurobehavioral functions and sleep physiology from chronic sleep restriction and total sleep deprivation. Sleep 26(2):117–126, 2003 12683469

Van Ham I, Verhoeven AA, Groenier KH, et al: Job satisfaction among general practitioners: a systematic literature review. Eur J Gen Pract 12(4):174–180, 2006 17127604

Waldinger RJ, Schulz MS: What's love got to do with it? Social functioning, perceived health, and daily happiness in married octogenarians. Psychol Aging 25(2):422–431, 2010 20545426

Weiner EL, Swain GR, Wolf B, Gottlieb M: A qualitative study of physicians' own wellness-promotion practices. West J Med 174(1):19–23, 2001 11154656

Whillans AV, Dunn EW, Smeets P, et al: Buying time promotes happiness. Proc Natl Acad Sci USA 114(32):8523–8527, 2017 28739889

Wise EH, Hersh MA, Gibson CM: Ethics, self-care and wellbeing for psychologists: reenvisioning the stress-distress continuum. Prof Psychol Res Pr 43(5):487–494, 2012

World Health Organization: Physical Activity Fact Sheet, 2018. Available at https://www.who.int/news-room/fact-sheets/detail/physical-activity. Accessed January 2, 2020.

CHAPTER 9

Mindfulness and Spiritual Well-Being

The real meditation practice is how we live our lives....

Jon Kabat-Zinn

Mindfulness has become a cultural buzzword in the past two decades, showing up in thousands of popular books, websites, and magazines, in addition to numerous scholarly articles. The effectiveness of mindfulness-based interventions for improving mental health and well-being, once considered to be a "fringe" therapeutic approach (Kabat-Zinn 2011), is now well documented. Meta-analysis has identified more than 200 empirical studies of mindfulness with overall moderate effect sizes in reducing psychopathology and improving well-being (Khoury et al. 2013). In certain areas, such as ameliorating anxiety and depression, effects have been even larger (Hofmann et al. 2010). For mental health clinicians, mindfulness practice offers a potential dual advantage of improving well-being for both clinicians and patients.

Mindfulness-Based Interventions

The term *mindfulness* is used to describe both a formal practice of meditation and a quality of being that can be brought to everyday life. Jon Kabat-Zinn, founder of mindfulness-based stress reduction (MBSR) and father of the mindfulness movement in psychotherapy, defined mindfulness as "paying attention in a particular way: on purpose, in the present moment, and nonjudgmentally" (Kabat-Zinn 1994, p. 4). Broadly, the umbrella term *mindfulness-based interventions* (MBIs) refers to an array of therapies that incorporate mindfulness. Several MBIs are well-researched programmatic psychotherapeutic approaches. Two of the most well-known MBIs, MBSR and mindfulness-based cognitive therapy, involve formal meditation. Several other well-studied approaches integrate less formal mindfulness: acceptance and commitment therapy, dialectical behavior therapy, and self-compassion and compassion-focused therapy.

Mindfulness-based approaches as a group represent the third wave of behavioral therapy treatment. In the earlier part of the twentieth century, behaviorism, the first wave, sought scientific objectivism and unbiased truth through observation and measurement in reaction to existing psychodynamic approaches. Behaviorism eliminated the individual's private experiences (i.e., thoughts and feelings). Instead, learning and conditioning were seen as a means to shift dysfunctional patterns of responding and targeted external behaviors.

Efforts to enhance efficacy, along with frustration with the focus on external behavior alone, led to a second wave of behavioral therapy treatment in the mid-twentieth century in which the focus shifted to internal experiences, specifically to thoughts. Cognitive-behavioral therapy (CBT) approaches posited that problem behaviors would decrease or be transformed following a change in dysfunctional and distorted thinking patterns (Hayes 2004). Although CBT is highly effective, a sizable number of patients do not respond to this treatment, and, overall, CBT does not outperform other approaches (Luborsky et al. 2006). The specificity of cognitive elements as the active change ingredient remains uncertain (see Hofmann and Asmundson 2008).

Aimed at addressing these limitations, mindfulness-based approaches developed under a third-wave shift in behaviorism. Mindfulness-based approaches differ from traditional CBT in their emphasis on *understanding* and altering the *functionality* of thoughts, feelings, and behaviors, as opposed to directly changing the *content* of these experiences (Hayes and Greco 2008). Resulting from the integration of Eastern philosophy into Western medical science, mindfulness-based approaches are sometimes viewed as an evolution of CBT, involving continued focus on internal experience with a new emphasis on how one relates to this experience and an emphasis on acceptance rather than change (Kabat-Zinn 2011).

Mindfulness and Wellness

Use of MBIs in psychiatry initially focused on the treatment of psychological distress and psychopathology; increasingly, the interest has been in using mindfulness to reduce global stress, increase self-compassion, and improve self-care (Shapiro and Carlson 2009). In sum, the goal is to enhance well-being. In fact, Kabat-Zinn (2011) originally conceived MBSR as a method for public health, as a solution to our overstimulated, fast-paced Western lifestyle in a digital age that leaves individuals increasingly out of touch with their sense of being, emotions, thoughts, and sensations. Walsh (2011) is one of many to argue that medicine ought to shift from an almost exclusive focus on the treatment of illness to a greater focus on helping patients develop healthy lifestyles. He counts mindfulness among these healthy lifestyle practices and cites "an explosion of meditation research" demonstrating "greater psychological, therapeutic, neural, physiological, biochemical, and chromosomal benefits…than are associated with any other psychotherapy" (Walsh 2011, p. 586).

Mindfulness for Mental Health Clinicians

Mindfulness is an excellent candidate for promotion of self-care among psychiatrists and psychologists for several reasons. First, the focus on wellness rather than pathology fits a growth mind-set, and the goal of improving satisfaction in the present moment is poised to combat the culture of overextension that leads to physician burnout. Second, mindfulness is associated with a host of outcomes that directly relate to interpersonal relationship elements in patient care, such as empathy and compassion, sensitivity, emotional stability, and psychological maturity (Shapiro and Carlson 2009). Third, mindfulness-based therapeutic approaches cannot be taught to patients soundly unless the clinician is a practitioner of mindfulness. As such, practicing mindfulness for self-care has a twofold benefit: enhancing physician well-being and improving clinical outcomes. For clinicians who struggle to put themselves first, learning and practicing mindfulness with the initial goal of helping better serve their patients can ultimately lead to learning to better attend to their own well-being needs.

MBSR is the most common way that physicians integrate mindfulness into treatments with their patients (Beach et al. 2013). MBSR is also the most widely studied programmatic approach in direct application for improving clinician well-being. A review paper by Irving et al. (2009) identified 10 studies of mindfulness training with medical students, nurses, physicians, psychologists, and counseling students aimed at improving clinician well-being. Across these studies, mindfulness training was shown to decrease depression, anxiety, burnout, stress, negative affect, and rumination and to increase empathy, self-compassion and compassion for others, spirituality, life satisfaction, and positive affect. Benefits were also seen for clinicians' patients: improved therapeutic relationships, greater ability to communicate and problem solve, and greater symptom improvement (Irving et al. 2009). It is important to note that the study sample sizes were small, and all but one lacked a comparison group. In the single controlled study, master's-level psychology students who completed eight sessions of MBSR reported significantly less stress, rumination, and anxiety, as well as increases in positive affect, self-compassion, and mindfulness, when compared with a wait-list control group of students who took another unrelated course (Shapiro et al. 2007). There were no randomized controlled trials (RCTs) among the 10 studies, and thus, mechanisms of action could not be identified.

Nevertheless, the promise of mindfulness for mental health professionals is appealing, given clear outcome of benefits across all studies and all provider degrees and specializations. Since that review, RCTs of the effects of mindfulness practice on medical student stress have been conducted, and outcomes have been positive (Warnecke et al. 2011). Additionally, a study in which psychotherapists-in-training were randomly assigned to use meditation prior to sessions demonstrated that their inpatient patients showed improvement in problem-solving, optimism, global severity of symptoms, specific anxiety, and psychosis scale ratings (Grepmair et al. 2007).

Combating Burnout and Enhancing Compassion With Mindfulness

Mindfulness has been shown to directly reduce burnout (Irving et al. 2009; Krasner et al. 2009; Shapiro and Carlson 2009) via improvements in provider self-care. Chaukos et al. (2017) found that residents who endorse burnout also have evidence of lower levels of mindfulness and coping skills. Loving-kindness and self-compassion are also closely linked to mindfulness, with some people arguing that mindfulness is a precursor for compassion toward the self and others. Klimecki and Singer (2012) argued that compassion toward others can prevent burnout because it allows for a connection with empathy in the present moment without the overinvolvement that results in personal distress. Research to date provides clear evidence that MBIs increase self-compassion (Boellinghaus et al. 2012), but it is less clear whether or not MBIs increase other types of compassion. Notably, professionals with lower self-compassion, those who are critical and controlling toward themselves, report less compassion toward their patients and demonstrate poorer patient outcomes (Henry et al. 1990).

Mindful Systems

With a highly burned-out and disillusioned workforce (roughly 50% of mental health professionals, as described in Chapter 3, "Burnout and Clinician Mental Health"), health care executives and administrative leaders face a considerable challenge (Shanafelt and Noseworthy 2017). Just as mindfulness can be an antidote to the burnout of an individual, a *system* that is mindful, aware, and values driven can combat burnout on a larger scale. As patients learn from the modeling and embodiment of healthy practices by professionals (Wise et al. 2012), clinicians can learn from the modeling and embodiment of a healthy system.

Organizationally, leaders and systems can embody the same elements of present-moment, sustained, nonjudgmental attention (Shanafelt and Noseworthy 2017). Crane and Ward (2016) suggest that *conscious leaders* look for small environmental changes to promote a culture of well-being, including intention to reward self-care, humorous books and jokes in the break room, and modeling of their own mindfulness practice. The incorporation of mindfulness practice into graduate and professional education and training (Wise et al. 2012) may have begun in order to promote self-care. As clinicians have shifted to a contemplative mind-set focusing on mindfulness and compassion, however, a wholesale shift in the culture of medicine has emerged. In the historical "us versus them" mentality, the invulnerable health care professional treated psychopathology in the vulnerable patient. Now, focusing on shared humanity, both the patient's and clinician's struggles are seen as an inevitable, yet surmountable, part of life. Described by Wise et al. (2012, p. 490) shared humanity is "an abiding acknowledgment of (providers) being truly human."

Religion and Spirituality

The focus of this chapter has been mindfulness as a way of being with self and others. The role of religion and prayer as a self-care practice also deserves note. It is estimated that 90% of the world's population engages in religious or spiritual practice, making religion almost universal (Koenig 2002). More than 700 studies have examined the impact of religious involvement on well-being, and more than half of these studies find positive associations, with increases in well-being, marital satisfaction, and life span, as well as reductions in anxiety, depression, substance abuse, and suicide. Authors note that religious or spiritual involvement is most likely to be beneficial when it centers on themes of love and forgiveness, themes that echo the core elements of mindfulness and self-compassion practices. In contrast, themes of punishment and guilt are predicted to have the opposite effect.

Participation in religious practice is confounded in the research with social support, community, and social service to others, all known predictors of well-being, making interpretations about the role of religious practice more challenging (Walsh 2011). The degree to which religious practice, as opposed to spiritual connection, enhances well-being is also unclear. Crane and Ward (2016) define *spiritual connection* as a sense of inner peace, a sense of purpose or place in the world, and a sense of trust that life will work out even when events are not understood. Avenues to spiritual connection include religious practice and prayer as well as contemplative practice, such as meditation or being absorbed in the beauty of nature. According to Crane and Ward, the goal of spiritual connection is to transcend and gain perspective on the challenges of daily life.

Connecting With Nature

Multiple studies have documented the restorative effects of natural environments (Berto 2014). Walsh (2011) notes that nature itself calms the nervous system and can enhance well-being, citing studies that find that hospital rooms with views of nature promote recovery, with patients evidencing less pain, better mood, better postsurgical outcomes, and shorter times to discharge. The existential benefits of nature can be used to support mindfulness. In comparison to the fast-paced digital world of *doing*, nature can provide a connection to simply *being*. Figure 9–1 shows simple actions that can bring more of the natural world into indoor spaces.

The Mindful Approach to Self-Care

Multiple avenues toward wellness and self-care are highlighted in this book. Mindfulness is unique in being not only a self-care practice but also a way in which to approach other self-care practices. Mindfulness can be used when interacting socially, eating, exercising, or even sleeping. Every action can be done nonjudgmentally, on purpose, in the present moment, with awareness. Mindfulness holds a great deal of promise

Sight

🌒 Hang up nature photos or artwork.
TIP: *Display photos that you have personally taken or artwork you have created yourself.*

🌒 Place plants thoughtfully around the indoor space.
CONSIDER *planting them yourself in containers you like.*

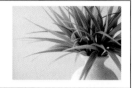

Sound

🌒 Listen to recordings of nature sounds.
CONSIDER *downloading an app that plays nature sounds on your phone.*

🌒 Listen to an indoor water fountain.
NOTICE *how you are feeling.*

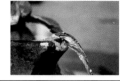

Smell

🌒 Fill the room with natural aromas through use of nature-scented essential oils or candles.
NOTICE *if these scents elicit any memories and then gently bring yourself back to the present moment.*

🌒 Keep flowers in the indoor space.
TIP: *Both freshly cut and dried flowers can offer lovely aromas.*

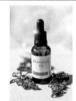

Taste

🌒 Engage in a mindful eating practice with a natural food.
CONSIDER *the journey this natural food item has taken to get from the ground to your taste buds.*

🌒 Sip a cup of herbal tea.
TIP: *Pick fresh herbs for your tea.*

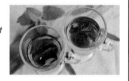

Touch

🌒 Plant an indoor container plant.
FEEL *the textures of the dirt, water, and plant.*

🌒 Open the window and feel the air and temperature on your skin.
FEEL *the sensations of a gust of wind or the heat of the sun.*

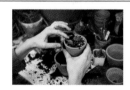

FIGURE 9–1. Bringing nature indoors.

Source. Reprinted from Carrión VG, Rettger J (eds): *Applied Mindfulness: Approaches in Mental Health for Children and Adolescents.* Washington, DC, American Psychiatric Association Publishing, 2019, p. 299. Copyright © 2019 American Psychiatric Association. Used with permission.

for mental health professionals in enhancing well-being. The positive practices in this chapter are intended to offer ways of infusing mindful living into a psychiatrist's or psychologist's existing schedule and life-style, without imposing more time-intensive demands. The following case example shows how one medical student incorporated mindfulness into his schedule.

Case Example

Lars David is a medical student in his final year. He has read about mindfulness-based approaches and is eager to integrate them into his patient care visits. He shares the benefits of mindfulness with his patients and encourages them to start a mindfulness practice. Although he is enthusiastic, he is unsure of how best to motivate his patients to use mindfulness. He notices that when he discusses mindfulness, his patients nod politely but show no signs of action. After attending a talk at grand rounds, Lars learns that mindfulness is difficult to teach or promote unless the teacher has an active personal practice. Lars makes the decision to begin to meditate daily and writes this on his to-do list. Week after week, he includes mindfulness on his daily to-dos but runs out of time meeting his demanding daily routine. With his long hours and intensive call schedule, fitting in an extra hour to meditate feels impossible.

A resident mentor shares with Lars that there is a small group of health care professionals who meet weekly for a seated and walking meditation. The group is open to all, operates on a drop-in basis, and requires no prior experience. Lars decides to attend. He quickly discovers that the practice of mindfulness is extremely challenging but also rewarding. Having a group of professionals with whom he can sit helps motivate Lars, and he appreciates the intimate connections he forms, even as a newcomer to the group. Lars is pleased to discover that the group is made up of both newbies like himself and seasoned practitioners. Even the seasoned practitioners share that the practice is often hard for them, that their minds wander, and that they must return their attention again and again to the object of their meditation. However, they also note that meditation has become easier with time and practice. Lars is encouraged to commit to regularly attending the group.

Contemplative traditions often inadvertently teach humility and directly break barriers between patient and clinician. Lars quickly discovers that instructing a patient to try mindfulness and sharing the joys and challenges of one's own mindfulness practice are entirely different. This scenario demonstrates the benefits of social support and a community of practicing health care professionals. A systemic culture in which mindfulness is part of a well-being practice promoted by the highest level of administration can enhance successful practice. In the absence of this, practitioners can still come together to form their own groups, regardless of their years of experience or expertise. Carving out time for self-care can quickly become another to-do for an already stressed health care professional, and Lars's situation suggests peer support as one antidote. Positive practices offered in the following section also focus on brief moments of mindfulness rather than daily seated practice. Importantly, brief moments of mindfulness are thought to be highly beneficial and worthwhile when longer formal practice is an unrealistic option.

Positive Practices

1. Take a few mornings to observe the first thing you do on waking up. Resist the urge to change it—just notice. Do you roll over in bed and silence your alarm? Do you leap up to begin your shower and start your day? Do you stumble to the kitchen to start the coffee? Is it the sound of someone else, perhaps a child needing attention, that kick-starts your day? Whatever it is, just observe. After observing for a few days, ask yourself if this way of starting the day feels good to you and is in line with your values. Finally, experiment with starting your morning in a more mindful manner. Open your eyes slowly. Stretch your arms slowly and fully above your head, savoring the sensation. Take a slow breath in and exhale it fully. Say a silent "good morning" in your head. Or conduct whatever other simple, slow, present-moment ritual feels right to you. Notice that this may have taken only 60 seconds to complete. Reflect on the experience.

2. Body scans are a common practice in MBSR and other mindfulness-based therapies. A traditional body scan walks the practitioner through every major body part via a guided practice that typically takes about 40 minutes to complete. This is an excellent pre-bedtime relaxation practice for anyone who struggles with insomnia or letting go of work-related thoughts and worries before falling asleep. Narrated body scans can easily be found for free online. Setting aside 40 minutes may feel daunting, particularly if you are new to mindfulness practice. However, body scans, like all mindfulness practices, can be simplified and shortened for the time that is available.

    The purpose of a body scan is simply to bring awareness to the body. Benefits of this awareness can include becoming more in touch with one's needs and internal sensations (e.g., hunger, fatigue, anxiety, neck tension, anger about a recent work meeting), gaining better understanding of oneself, and relaxing. Relaxation is not the goal of a body scan per se. If you become aware of annoyance in the body after completing a body scan, for example, the exercise has still been done correctly. Annoyance may be an unpleasant sensation, but its presence may point to something bothersome in life or something that has been suppressed. Awareness and exploration of annoyance may lead to problem-solving about an unresolved issue.

For an abbreviated body scan, select as many or as few body parts as desired. Conduct the body scan lying down, seated, or standing, in the peace and comfort of a private office or in the midst of the bustle of a meeting, rounds, or a therapy session. Simply bring awareness to the feet, noticing sensation in the toes, arch, and the top of the foot. Rest attention on the feet for 20 seconds, then move awareness to the legs. Continue scanning up the body, exploring the seat, abdomen, chest, shoulders, arms, neck, and head. If time is limited, simply practice grounding awareness for a few seconds on one body part.

3. Mindfulness often begins with the breath. The goal is not to change the breath but simply to notice it. Many people struggle when attempting to engage in meditation. Focusing on the breath is a great way to ease in, and typically, the biggest challenge is remembering to practice. New habits are easier to create when made very small and paired with already learned behaviors. Practitioners often find it helpful to pair a mindful breath with a semifrequently completed activity, such as answering the phone. Each time the phone rings or before initiating a phone call, use the ringing or lifting of the phone as a cue to take a full, deep, mindful breath. Other cues might include walking through a doorway, coming to a red light while driving, or placing your hands over the keyboard to initiate typing. Be creative in generating mindful breath cues. But resist the urge to overdo it— try to pick just one stimulus to start.

4. Many people eat at their desks or in a meeting, cram in a protein bar or other portable food on the go, or maybe miss lunch altogether. Instead, try even once per week to take a full lunch break. If this seems like an impossibility, take note! Resist the urge to rationalize this behavior ("no one else takes lunch either"). Instead, be appropriately appalled. Everyone deserves a lunch break, and it is incredible that this attitude persists. Perhaps it is time to simply notice your behavior and say compassionately to yourself, "Wow, my body works so hard. It is hard to allocate time to take care of it. Right now, my body is not permitted to take a break to refuel." Compassionately feel any regret or sadness that may arise.

If you do take lunch, thank yourself for this self-care gift and move on to a mindful eating exercise. This can involve a silent lunch with yourself, in which you do not work, read, listen to music, talk to colleagues, or otherwise do anything except eat. Allow yourself to fully involve all of your senses as you observe the colors on your plate, feel the textures on your tongue, inhale the aroma through your nostrils, and savor the flavors. You can even listen to the joyful crunch of fresh food. If your food is not so fresh or delicious, allow for this awareness. Try not to judge yourself; simply notice.

5. Find a few minutes in your day to go outside. On days when your schedule allows, this could involve going for a walk—perhaps alone, perhaps with a colleague. You might even propose turning a traditional meeting into a walking meeting, in which business is conducted as you stroll outside. If appropriate, stash a more comfortable pair of shoes at the office in anticipation of going outside. When your schedule does not permit even a brief walk, merely stepping outside for 2 minutes, breathing in fresh air, stretching your arms overhead, and taking stock of the weather with a slow and present gaze can be beneficial.

Conclusion

Mindfulness practices predict a host of beneficial outcomes, including reductions in anxiety and depressed mood as well as enhanced empathy, compassion, and general well-being. Further, mindfulness has been found to be a powerful antidote to burnout. As a self-care practice, mindfulness has the dual advantage of directly benefiting both the clinician and the patient. Patients report both reduction in psychiatric symptoms and increased well-being and warmth in the therapeutic relationship when their clinicians practice mindfulness. To offer effective and authentic mindfulness interventions to patients, clinicians need to have some type of regular experiential practice. Embracing mindfulness does not require a huge time commitment to daily seated practice, however; even briefly applied practice in daily life has been shown to have enormous benefit.

Exercises

—————O—————

1. **Wherever you are, take a moment to notice your surroundings.** What do you hear? What do you see? What can you smell or feel? Keep a nonjudgmental attitude and just observe. Write down your observations.

—————————————————————

—————————————————————

—————————————————————

2. Write down three activities you could practice doing mindfully this week.

_____

_____

_____

3. Consider what you could do to add more exposure to nature into your day.

_____

_____

_____

———————O———————

Recommended Resources

Brach T: Radical Acceptance: Embracing Your Life With the Heart of a Buddha. New York, Bantam, 2004

Kabat-Zinn J: Full Catastrophe Living: Using the Wisdom of Your Body and Mind to Face Stress, Pain, and Illness, Revised Edition. New York, Bantam, 2013

Neff K: Self-Compassion: The Proven Power of Being Kind to Yourself. New York, Harper Collins, 2011

Noordsy DL (ed): Lifestyle Psychiatry. Washington, DC, American Psychiatric Association Publishing, 2019

Shapiro S, White C: Mindful Discipline: A Loving Approach to Setting Limits and Raising an Emotionally Intelligent Child. Oakland, CA, New Harbinger, 2014

Zerbo E, Schlechter A, Desai S, Levounis P: Becoming Mindful: Integrating Mindfulness Into Your Psychiatric Practice. Arlington, VA, American Psychiatric Association Publishing, 2016

References

Beach MC, Roter D, Korthuis PT, et al: A multicenter study of physician mindfulness and health care quality. Ann Fam Med 11(5):421–428, 2013 24019273

Berto R: The role of nature in coping with psycho-physiological stress: a literature review on restorativeness. Behav Sci (Basel) 4(4):394–409, 2014 25431444

Boellinghaus I, Jones FW, Hutton J: The role of mindfulness and loving kindness meditation in cultivating self-compassion and other-focused concern in health care professionals. Mindfulness 5(2):129–138, 2012

Chaukos D, Chad-Friedman E, Mehta DH, et al: Risk and resilience factors associated with resident burnout. Acad Psychiatry 41(2):189–194, 2017 28028738

Crane PJ, Ward SF: Self-healing and self-care for nurses. AORN J 104(5):386–400, 2016 27793249

Grepmair L, Mitterlehner F, Loew T, et al: Promoting mindfulness in psychotherapists in training influences the treatment results of their patients: a randomized, double-blind, controlled study. Psychother Psychosom 76:332–338, 2007 17917468

Hayes SC: Acceptance and commitment therapy, relational frame theory, and the third wave of behavioral and cognitive therapies. Behav Ther 35(4):639–665, 2004

Hayes S, Greco L: Acceptance and mindfulness for youth: it's time, in Acceptance and Mindfulness Treatments for Children and Adolescents: A Practitioner's Guide. Edited by Greco LA, Hayes SC. Oakland, CA, New Harbinger, 2008, pp 3–13

Henry WP, Schacht TE, Strupp HH: Patient and therapist introject, interpersonal process, and differential psychotherapy outcome. J Consult Clin Psychol 58(6):768–774, 1990 2292626

Hofmann SG, Asmundson GJG: Acceptance and mindfulness-based therapy: new wave or old hat? Clin Psychol Rev 28(1):1–16, 2008 17904260

Hofmann SG, Sawyer AT, Witt AA, Oh D: The effect of mindfulness-based therapy on anxiety and depression: a meta-analytic review. J Consult Clin Psychol 78(2):169–183, 2010 20350028

Irving JA, Dobkin PL, Park J: Cultivating mindfulness in health care professionals: a review of empirical studies of mindfulness-based stress reduction (MBSR). Complement Ther Clin Pract 15(2):61–66, 2009 19341981

Kabat-Zinn J: Wherever You Go, There You Are: Mindfulness Meditation in Everyday Life. New York, Hyperion, 1994

Kabat-Zinn J: Some reflections on the origins of MBSR, skillful means, and the trouble with maps. Contemp Buddhism 12(1):281–300, 2011

Khoury B, Lecomte T, Fortin G, et al: Mindfulness-based therapy: a comprehensive meta-analysis. Clin Psychol Rev 33(6):763–771, 2013 23796855

Klimecki O, Singer T: Empathic distress fatigue rather than compassion fatigue? Integrating findings from empathy research in psychology and social neuroscience, in Pathological Altruism. Edited by Oakley B, Knafo A, Madhavan G, Wilson DS. New York, Oxford University Press, 2012, pp 368–383

Koenig HG: Religion, congestive heart failure, and chronic pulmonary disease. J Relig Health 41(3):263–278, 2002

Krasner MS, Epstein RM, Beckman H, et al: Association of an educational program in mindful communication with burnout, empathy, and attitudes among primary care physicians. JAMA 302(12):1284–1293, 2009 19773563

Luborsky L, Rosenthal R, Diguer L, et al: The dodo bird verdict is alive and well—mostly. Clin Psychol Sci Pract 9(1):2–12, 2006

Shanafelt TD, Noseworthy JH: Executive leadership and physician well-being: nine organizational strategies to promote engagement and reduce burnout. Mayo Clin Proc 92(1):129–146, 2017 27871627

Shapiro SL, Carlson LE: The Art and Science of Mindfulness: Integrating Mindfulness Into Psychology and the Helping Professions. Washington, DC, American Psychological Association, 2009

Shapiro SL, Brown KW, Biegel GM: Teaching self-care to caregivers: effects of mindfulness-based stress reduction on the mental health of therapists in training. Training and Education in Professional Psychology 1(2):105–115, 2007

Walsh R: Lifestyle and mental health. Am Psychol 66(7):579–592, 2011 21244124

Warnecke E, Quinn S, Ogden K, et al: A randomised controlled trial of the effects of mindfulness practice on medical student stress levels. Med Educ 45(4):381–388, 2011 21401686

Wise EH, Hersch MA, Gibson CM: Ethics, self-care and well-being for psychologists: reenvisioning the stress-distress continuum. Prof Psychol Res Pr 43(5):487–494, 2012

CHAPTER 10

Nutrition and Physical Activity

In years past, a favorite pearl of wisdom for medical students and residents in the very earliest stages of training was "Eat when you can, sleep when you must." This message stated, explicitly, that proper sleep, healthy nutrition, and balanced physical activity were a low priority and that the ability to ignore the needs of the body was, in fact, a badge of honor.

For anyone working in mental health, the day-to-day challenges of balancing clinical work, research, and administrative responsibilities with family obligations are obvious. These challenges are compounded by stresses inherent to the mental health field, such as bearing witness to emotional stories, managing boundaries, and dealing with poor outcomes or disgruntled patients and families. Stressed individuals may find it more difficult to care for themselves and may turn to comfort eating, consumption of alcohol, or neglect of the physical body.

Clinician self-care, including nutrition and physical activity, is of paramount importance. Studies have documented correlations between physicians' health behaviors and their interactions with patients about said behaviors (Abramson et al. 2000; Frank et al. 2010). Moreover, self-care has been deemed an area of core competency by some physician practice governing bodies (Frank 2005). In this chapter, we not only review the notable nutrition and physical activity health behaviors for the mental health care professional but also discuss practical individual-level, as well as institution-wide, practices to best support, invest in, and promote the wellness behaviors of clinicians.

Nutrition

Proper nutrition is essential for promoting optimal health and well-being for everyone, regardless of profession. The "hangry" phenomenon popularized by the Snickers candy bar commercials over the past few years has become a common experience. When people are hungry, they are not themselves. They can be irritable, lose patience, get easily annoyed, and have trouble with concentration and focus. Clinical experience with patients living with eating disorders demonstrates this even further. Individuals with anorexia nervosa, bulimia nervosa, and binge eating disorders describe signs and symptoms of malnutrition that may mimic the neurovegetative symptoms of depression (Keys et al. 1950). These symptoms include problems with sleeping (either insomnia or hypersomnia), anhedonia, low energy, social isolation, social withdrawal, anxiety, and impaired concentration and poor focus that can lead to the perception of impaired cognitive function and to difficulties with increased stress across life domains (e.g., relationships, work, hobbies). Severe starvation dramatically affects clarity of thought and sustained mental effort. In fact, imaging studies of the brains of individuals with anorexia nervosa consistently show decreased volumes of white matter that are reversible with proper renourishment (Wagner et al. 2006).

Undereating due to stress is problematic. So, too, are patterns of overeating. When particularly busy, or fueled by morning coffee or tea, many individuals note that they do not feel hungry. They are not attuned to hunger cues and do not necessarily realize that their bodies are in need of nutrition, leading to skipped meals. Not until they get home do these individuals notice that they are, in fact, quite hungry. This often leads to overconsumption of calories within a relatively short period of time, with the individual rationalizing this behavior as permissible because he or she did not eat breakfast or lunch. The individual might have thoughts such as "I have been 'good' all day, so it is OK to overeat now." Patterns of restrictive eating followed by binge eating are particularly problematic in that they are associated with weight gain, morbidity, and mortality, stemming from resultant insulin resistance, dyslipidemia, hypertension, and cardiac disease (Olguin et al. 2017).

People living in larger bodies may need to contend with the emotional stress that results from weight stigma (Romano et al. 2018). Individuals of all sizes may be motivated to start overly restrictive eating or exercise plans designed for weight loss that may result in ongoing unhealthy eating patterns. People may also struggle to maintain regular, healthy nutrition practices when trying to function in stressful situations. It may be helpful to consult the 2015–2020 Dietary Guidelines for Americans of the U.S. Department of Health and Human Services and the U.S. Department of Agriculture, which can be downloaded at http://health.gov/dietaryguidelines/2015/guidelines. The guidelines recommend following a healthy eating pattern that includes a variety of vegetables, fruits, grains, fat-free or low-fat dairy (and/or fortified soy beverages), proteins, and oils, while limiting saturated and trans fats, added sugars, and sodium (U.S. Department of Health and Human Services and U.S. Department of Agriculture 2015).

Physical Activity

Physical activity provides various and substantial positive impacts on both physical and psychological well-being. Indeed, regular physical activity can contribute to reduced risk of developing chronic diseases such as obesity, diabetes, and certain types of cancer, as well as other health problems. Additional health concerns include hypertension, coronary heart disease, and cardiac arrest (U.S. Department of Health and Human Services [USDHHS] 2018). Regular physical activity works to prevent and reduce obesity onset via increase in energy expenditure and lean muscle and a simultaneous decrease in body fat percentage (Blair and Holder 2002). Consistent physical activity has been documented as a critical contributor to successful weight loss maintenance (USDHHS 2018). Weight-bearing exercises in particular offer additional benefits of assisting adults to reach and sustain peak bone mass. Table 10–1 outlines sample activities organized by intensity level.

The psychological benefits of physical activity are significant and include improved mood and reduction of anxiety and stress (Task Force on Community Preventive Services 2002; USDHHS 2018). Reviews of decades' worth of research on the impact of physical activity on depression highlight the benefits of exercise as both prevention and treatment for subclinical and full-syndrome depressive episodes (Rebar et al. 2015; Schuch et al. 2016; Takács 2014). Exercise guidelines for adults suggest the following (USDHHS 2018):

- Move more and sit less every day.
- Engage in moderate (e.g., brisk walking) and vigorous (e.g., running, lap swimming) activity for optimal health benefits.
  - Aim for 2.5–5 hours of moderate activity every week.
  - Aim for 1.25–2.5 hours of vigorous activity every week.
  - Spread this aerobic physical activity throughout the week.

TABLE 10–1. Examples of activities by intensity level

Moderate-intensity activities
- Walking briskly (2.5 miles per hour or faster)
- Recreational swimming
- Bicycling slower than 10 miles per hour on level terrain
- Tennis (doubles)
- Active forms of yoga (e.g., Vinyasa or power yoga)
- Ballroom or line dancing
- General yard work and home repair work
- Exercise classes like water aerobics

Vigorous-intensity exercises
- Jogging or running
- Swimming laps
- Tennis (singles)
- Vigorous dancing
- Bicycling faster than 10 miles per hour
- Jumping rope
- Heavy yard work (digging or shoveling, with heart rate increases)
- Hiking uphill or with a heavy backpack
- High-intensity interval training (HIIT)
- Exercise classes like vigorous step aerobics or kickboxing

Source. Reprinted from U.S. Department of Health and Human Services: Physical Activity Guidelines for Americans, 2nd Edition. Washington, DC, U.S. Department of Health and Human Services, 2018. Available at: https://health.gov/paguidelines/second-edition/pdf/Physical_Activity_Guidelines_2nd_edition.pdf. Accessed July 23, 2019.

- Engage in strength training for additional benefits.
  - Aim to exercise 2 or more days every week.
  - Use all major muscle groups.

Nutrition and Physical Activity Behaviors Among Physicians

Research on the nutrition and physical activity health behaviors of physicians is informative. One study demonstrated that the physical activity behaviors of medical students decreased throughout their years of training (Frank et al. 2006). Another study found that only 21% of physicians surveyed were achieving 30 minutes of moderate activity each week (Gupta and Fan 2009). Most clinicians cited insufficient time and lack of workout facilities and motivation as contributors.

Case Example

Satvik Kumar has been in practice for 20 years. In training, he prided himself on prioritizing clinical care above all else and frequently received positive feedback from his preceptors and rotation directors about his discipline and devotion. Since starting his busy psychiatry practice, Dr. Kumar has tried his best to balance the demands of patient care and administrative work with his desire to be present in his relationship and attentive to the needs of his children. Although he was previously athletic and used to run 5K charity races on the weekend with his friends, running and exercising have largely fallen by the wayside. He does not have time to train any longer and feels that he is far too out of shape to run a race. In fact, he has gained approximately 25 pounds since he finished his residency.

When he wakes up in the morning, Dr. Kumar hits the snooze button more times than he had planned and has time only for a cup of coffee as he rushes out the door. He has another cup of coffee as he enters the office and usually works through lunch, returning patient phone calls, completing charting, or responding to text messages from his partner or children. He generally feels exhausted by the end of the day and works hard to avoid snapping at office staff when they ask questions.

When Dr. Kumar returns home in the early evening, he has fallen into the habit of snacking while watching the news and chatting with his partner. He snacks on cheese and crackers, nuts, or chips while they come up with a dinner plan. Because they both work full-time, they often rely on frozen dinners or prepared meals or order takeout delivery. They also often attend evening activities, so they usually eat quickly. Sometimes they eat while standing at the kitchen counter or while using social media on their cell phones. Dr. Kumar typically spends the remainder of the evening helping his children with homework or attending school sports activities, and he often has a snack with his kids before their bedtime in order to increase their time spent together. He tries to read a few pages of a novel before bed while enjoying a glass of wine. Inevitably, he complains to his partner that he has indigestion and feels too full, and he commits to trying to be "healthier" the following day.

Dr. Kumar's employer introduces a new wellness initiative, making it a good and timely opportunity to start healthy changes. Dr. Kumar has an opportunity to meet with a coach to put his commitment to being healthy into action. His initial thought is that he needs a complete overhaul of his behaviors and states that he wants to eat healthy and exercise every day. The wellness coach asks him to complete an assessment of his nutrition and exercise behaviors and honestly rate his motivation for change. She also encourages him to be realistic about goal setting and to break down his goals into smaller and more manageable pieces.

Dr. Kumar agrees that he is more likely to be consistent with behavior change if he can tackle one issue at a time and have some accountability. He enlists his partner for help, and they decide that they will first focus on making sure to eat breakfast daily. They find recipes, such as overnight oats or individual egg bites, that they can batch cook together on weekends and then have available for breakfast during the workweek. They also purchase granola bars and fruit to keep in the car and office so that healthy eating options are available even when life becomes too busy. Dr. Kumar makes a promise to eat breakfast at home with the family at least 3 days each week and makes an appointment to follow up with the wellness coach 2 weeks later to chart his progress.

At the 2-week check-in, Dr. Kumar reports that the family has been eating breakfast together most days and that his kids have been excited to participate in choosing recipes and cooking as a family. He feels more energetic and resilient during the workday and no longer craves a glass of wine before bed. He missed breakfast once when car trouble threw him off schedule, but he was able to eat a granola bar and apple while he finished morning paperwork. The coach talks with him about maintaining his new behavior change, and Dr. Kumar feels motivated to start bringing leftovers from the night before to make sure he has a proper lunch each day. He wants to make a plan to start running again at his next wellness coaching appointment.

Dr. Kumar's situation is all too familiar to busy clinicians. Balancing work-related tasks with running a household, caring for children, and nurturing a relationship can feel overwhelming. It often feels as though there is not enough time in the day to prioritize regular exercise or prepare healthy meals. It is, however, far easier to stay on top of competing responsibilities when one is adequately nourished and refreshed. Otherwise, it is easy to slip into patterns of overeating (or undereating), sedentary living, and overconsumption of alcohol.

When setting goals for making behavioral change, it is important to make them specific, measurable, and achievable. It helps considerably to enlist friends or significant others to maintain accountability, to develop back-up plans in the event of an unforeseen conflict, and to practice self-compassion when life does not go exactly as planned. The ability to consult with a coach who has experience with helping people set manageable and achievable goals is an added bonus and is becoming increasingly available through workplace wellness programs.

Institutional Support

There are steps that institutions can take to help advocate for and support their staff effectively. First, institutions should be held responsible for creating and cultivating a culture of self-care. The myth that never-ill doctors are available round the clock to put others' needs before their own fundamental self-care must be dispelled. Many institutions have thoughtfully revamped hospital cafeterias to include a wider variety of fresh and healthy options. A number of systems have incorporated wellness programs that provide financial incentives for employees to complete wellness assessments (including an evaluation of nutrition habits and measurement of physical characteristics, such as weight and cholesterol), attend classes on nutrition, or work with a consultant to set nutrition goals. Some academic medicine departments, such as Stanford's Emergency Medicine Department (Fassiotto et al. 2018), have experimented with offering credits for a meal kit delivery so that physicians do not need to contend with the challenges of grocery shopping and meal preparation at the end of a stressful day. The British Columbia Medical Association implements an annual Walk With Your Doc Initiative (British Columbia Medical Association 2019). In 2012, the event was attended by 1,000 physicians and 2,000 patients. This event represents a simple way large, well-respected institutions can advocate and support health for both physicians and patients. The National Alliance on Mental Illness also orchestrates an annual walk for people affected by mental illness, including patients and their families, clinicians, health care system administrative staff, and more (www.namiwalks.org). Events sponsored by institutions demonstrate their advocacy of such work and create a community around participation and personal expression. Other simple ways to augment physical activity throughout the institution include turning mentorship meetings into walking meetings, developing the opportunity for lunchtime yoga, and installing additional bike racks in front of the office and clinical buildings.

Positive Practices

Nutrition

1. Prioritize mealtimes. Devote at least a few minutes to eating your meal away from your desk, if possible, rather than trying to multitask. Try to eat with colleagues or video chat with a friend or family member to encourage conversation. Use real plates and flatware to make mealtime a more pleasant experience.

2. If you know that there are certain times of the day that you are vulnerable for poor food choices, seek added support or structure during those times. For example, if you tend to dive into a bag of chips after work, have healthier options at the ready. Ask your significant other or a friend for support. Or engage in an activity that is soothing and keeps your hands busy, such as working a puzzle, knitting, or drawing. If you still feel a hankering for chips, allow yourself to have them without judgment and try to mindfully determine when you are satisfied or satiated. If your tendency is to undereat, ask friends and family for reminders and support. Resist the urge to skip meals when feeling busy or stressed.

3. If you feel you need education about how to consume a balanced diet, consult with a dietitian. Be realistic and reasonable in nutrition planning. For example, do not pledge to bring lunch every day if you have never done so before. It is important to set SMART goals, that is, goals that are specific, measurable, achievable, realistic, and timely. A more reasonable place to start is to make a goal of bringing your lunch 2 days per week and to bring lunch on days when you have cooked meals the night before that reliably produce leftovers. You can troubleshoot challenges and successes at the end of the week and make adjustments based on what you have learned. Also, keep in mind that it can take a full month or more to implement a new habit.

4. Remember that a slip does not mean you are back to square one. If a meal or snack does not go as planned, let it go and try again at the next meal or snack. People get in trouble when they have an "all or nothing" mentality: "I overate already today. I might as well just eat what I want and try again tomorrow."

Physical Activity

1. Be sure to engage in a physical activity you enjoy. Research shows that people are more likely to repeat activities they find enjoyable. Adding music or a podcast to workouts or being outdoors in an aesthetically pleasing environment can help infuse enjoyment.

2. Participate in an activity you feel confident about and have mastered.

Conclusion

For both professional effectiveness and quality of life, taking care of the physical body is critical. Although psychiatrists and psychologists face many work and life demands that can make healthy eating and regular physical activity challenging to achieve, both immediate and long-term psychological and physical health outcomes depend on adequate nutrition and exercise. Starting with a self-care mind-set can help. Psychiatrists and psychologists can consider their own values and make a commitment to prioritizing the healthy actions that are important to them personally. Building a network of like-minded individuals who provide accountability and support can also contribute to the joy of doing what is good for oneself. Finally, within health care systems, encouraging, scaffolding, and rewarding clinicians' self-care practices can translate into healthy professionals as well as optimal patient care.

Exercises

———————o———————

1. **Practice self-compassion.** If you overeat or undereat, notice and be curious about why, without judgment. For example, "I seem to be gravitating toward a lot of comfort foods and wine lately. I wonder what that is about. Maybe I am feeling more stressed with this quality improvement project than I initially thought."

   Write down what you notice here.

   _____

   _____

   _____

   If you rely on food during stressful times, what other methods could you use to deal with stress?

   _____

   _____

   _____

2. **Pay attention to food.** Try to eat regular meals and snacks over the course of the day. It can be helpful to keep a food log like the one below to notice patterns in eating. It is usu-

ally best to eat every 3–4 hours if possible. This makes it less likely that you will have urges to engage in binge eating (typically triggered by the triad of hunger, stress, and limited identified coping strategies). Be aware of alcohol consumption because this can add additional calories and also can promote overeating.

	Mon.	Tues.	Wed.	Thurs.	Fri	Sat.	Sun.
Breakfast:							
(A.M. snacks)							
Lunch:							
(P.M. snacks)							
Dinner:							
(Other)							

3. **Have a fallback plan.** If you oversleep and do not have time for breakfast at home, be sure to have a stash of nutrition bars, dried fruit, or nuts available in the car or at the office. If there is a fast food restaurant on the way, take note of healthier options that you may take advantage of in an urgent situation. Keep healthy and satisfying snacks at the ready.

    What are the times when you are most likely to have problems sticking to a healthy diet?

    _____

    _____

    _____

    What can you do to be better prepared for these issues in advance?

    _____

    _____

    _____

4. **Enlist support.** Get colleagues, friends, and/or family members to participate in activities with you. Social support can play a helpful role in the initiation and sustainability of physical activity (Lindsay Smith et al. 2017; Rackow et al. 2015).

   Make a list here of people who could support your efforts to get more exercise.

   _____

   _____

   _____

5. **Self-monitor.** Tracking your physical activities behaviors (e.g., with a Fitbit, smartphone health application, basic pedometer) can help motivate you. Write here how you will monitor your physical activity.

   _____

   _____

   _____

———————O———————

Recommended Resources

Albers S: Eating Mindfully: How to End Mindless Eating and Enjoy a Balanced Relationship with Food. Oakland, CA, New Harbinger, 2012

Hahn TN, Cheung L: Savor: Mindful Eating, Mindful Life. New York, HarperCollins, 2010

Kimiecik J: The Intrinsic Exerciser: Discovering the Joy of Exercise. New York, Houghton Mifflin, 2002

Noordsy DL (ed): Lifestyle Psychiatry. Washington, DC, American Psychiatric Association Publishing, 2019

Suzuki W: The brain-changing benefits of exercise (video). TEDWomen, 2017. Available at: www.ted.com/talks/wendy_suzuki_the_brain_changing_benefits_of_exercise/up-next?language=en. Accessed December 12, 2019.

Suzuki W, Fitzpatrick B: Healthy Brain, Happy Life: A Personal Program to Activate Your Brain and Do Everything Better. New York, HarperCollins, 2015

References

Abramson S, Stein J, Schaufele M, et al: Personal exercise habits and counseling practices of primary care physicians: a national survey. Clin J Sport Med 10(1):40–48, 2000 10695849

Blair SN, Holder S: Exercise in the management of obesity, in Eating Disorders and Obesity: A Comprehensive Handbook. Edited by Fairburn CG, Brownell KD. New York, Guilford, 2002, pp 518–523

British Columbia Medical Association: Walk with your doc. Available at: https://walkwithyourdoc.ca. Accessed April 25, 2019.

Fassiotto M, Simard C, Sandborg C, et al: An integrated career coaching and time-banking system promoting flexibility, wellness, and success: a pilot program at Stanford University School of Medicine. Acad Med 93(6):881–887, 2018 29298183

Frank E, Carrera JS, Elon L, Hertzberg VS: Basic demographics, health practices, and health status of U.S. medical students. Am J Prev Med 31(6):499–505, 2006 17169711

Frank E, Segura C, Shen H, Oberg E: Predictors of Canadian physicians' prevention counseling practices. Can J Public Health 101(5):390–395, 2010 21214054

Frank JR (ed): The CanMEDS 2005 Physician Competency Framework. Ottawa, ON, Canada, Royal College of Physicians and Surgeons of Canada, 2005

Gupta K, Fan L: Doctors: fighting fit or couch potatoes? Br J Sports Med 43(2):153–154, 2009 19050002

Keys A, Brozek J, Henschel A, et al: The Biology of Human Starvation. Minneapolis, University of Minnesota Press, 1950

Lindsay Smith G, Banting L, Eime R, et al: The association between social support and physical activity in older adults: a systematic review. Int J Behav Nutr Phys Act 14(1):56, 2017 28449673

Olguin P, Fuentes M, Gabler G, et al: Medical comorbidity of binge eating disorder. Eat Weight Disord 22(1):13–26, 2017 27553016

Rackow P, Scholz U, Hornung R: Received social support and exercising: an intervention study to test the enabling hypothesis. Br J Health Psychol 20(4):763–776, 2015 25854295

Rebar AL, Stanton R, Geard D, et al: A meta-meta-analysis of the effect of physical activity on depression and anxiety in non-clinical adult populations. Health Psychol Rev 9(3):366–378, 2015 25739893

Romano E, Haynes A, Robinson E: Weight perception, weight stigma concerns, and overeating. Obesity (Silver Spring) 26(8):1365–1371, 2018 29956497

Schuch FB, Vancampfort D, Richards J, et al: Exercise as a treatment for depression: a meta-analysis adjusting for publication bias. J Psychiatr Res 77:42–51, 2016 26978184

Takács J: Regular physical activity and mental health: the role of exercise in the prevention of, and intervention in depressive disorders [in Hungarian]. Psychiatr Hung 29(4):386–397, 2014 25569828

Task Force on Community Preventive Services: Recommendations to increase physical activity in communities. Am J Prev Med 22(4)(suppl):67–72, 2002 11985935

U.S. Department of Health and Human Services: Physical Activity Guidelines for Americans, 2nd Edition. Washington, DC, U.S. Department of Health and Human Services, 2018

U.S. Department of Health and Human Services and U.S. Department of Agriculture: Dietary Guidelines for Americans 2015–2020, 8th Edition. Washington, DC, U.S. Department of Health and Human Services, December 2015. Available at: http://health.gov/dietaryguidelines/2015/guidelines. Accessed July 16, 2019.

Wagner A, Greer P, Bailer UF, et al: Normal brain tissue volumes after long-term recovery in anorexia and bulimia nervosa. Biol Psychiatry 59(3):291–293, 2006 16139807

ॐ✖

CHAPTER 11

Sleep

It is a common experience that a problem difficult at night is resolved in the morning after the committee of sleep has worked on it.

John Steinbeck

A solid night's sleep can make a world of difference when it comes to optimal function during the day. Yet, as basic and essential as it is, sleep is often the first activity to go when life gets busy. Whether completing documentation, taking hospital or emergency department calls, or caring for infants and small children, mental health professionals are prone to sacrificing sleep to meet competing demands from their professional and personal lives. To compensate for these job and home life pressures, mental health professionals may feel obliged to stay up late at night or wake up early in the morning, adding more time to an already busy day. In the long term, this strategy may lead to burnout and an increased risk for negative health consequences. Professionals may even develop diagnosable sleep disorders, further exacerbating the challenges of juggling work and home life demands.

Recent studies by the U.S. Centers for Disease Control and Prevention indicate that approximately 35% of adults sleep fewer than 7 hours each night (Liu et al. 2016). Some well-known personalities claim to get by with only 4 hours of sleep per night; others do best with more than 10 hours nightly. The National Sleep Foundation recommends that adults have 7–9 hours of sleep each night to function optimally (Hirshkowitz et al. 2015).

Benefits of Sleep

Why is sleep so important? Sleep is homeostatically protected across species despite the fact that organisms are vulnerable when they are not alert. Sleep serves an essential purpose. Laboratory animal studies show that extended sleep deprivation can result in death (Rechtschaffen and Bergmann 1995). For humans, both patterns of excessive sleep and patterns of sleep deprivation are linked with heightened mortality risk (Ferrie et al. 2007; Tamakoshi et al. 2004). Although psychiatrists and psychologists do not currently understand every nuanced function of sleep, current thinking suggests that the brain uses sleep to allow the body to rest, repair, and rejuvenate—essentially to "clean up" and process the events of the day. Learning is consolidated and memory is laid down (Maier and Nissen 2017). People consistently perform better on cognitive measures when allowed to sleep longer the night before (Boardman et al. 2018). Adults who have less than the recommended amount of sleep each night have a higher risk of insulin resistance, diabetes, and heart disease (Liu et al. 2016).

Without good sleep, both ability to function and to work productivity suffer. Attention and affect regulation also suffer when individuals have inadequate sleep, because of either complete sleep deprivation for an acute period or chronic partial sleep deprivation (Krause et al. 2017). Medical errors are more common among sleep-deprived physicians (Olson et al. 2009). Patients treated by physicians who are sleep deprived may be at slightly greater risk of complications (Rothschild et al. 2009). Additionally, sleep-deprived individuals may not be fully aware of their deficits in this state (Harrison and Horne 2000). The following vignette provides an example of one clinician's struggle to balance sleep needs with his personal and professional aspirations.

Vignette

Brian Song, age 60, has never previously had any difficulties with sleep. In the last year, he has had trouble falling and staying asleep each night and is frequently sleepy during the day. He used to retire around 10 P.M. each night and wake at 6 A.M. After hearing about many prominent figures being able to function on 4–6 hours of sleep each night, he decided to stay up until midnight instead. He was motivated by his desire to work on a book that he has always wanted to write, but, previously, he had been unwilling to take time away from his wife and children. He felt that sleeping less "just makes sense."

Since he started a new sleeping schedule 8 months ago, Dr. Song reports that he has felt mildly irritable with his family and staff but is able to remain calm and professional with the patients he treats. He has gone from drinking a cup of herbal tea each morning to drinking a cup of coffee before leaving the house each morning. He has another coffee on his train ride to the hospital, when he generally reads the newspaper. He frequently finds himself nodding off during his commute, and once he was surprised and embarrassed to be awakened by the conductor when he missed his stop and rode to the end of the line. Dr. Song is reluctant to change his schedule, however, because he enjoys being productive when everyone else in the house is asleep and hopes he will be ready to shop a draft of his book in the coming months.

When his yearly physical is due, his wife suggests that he talk with his doctor about his sleep needs. Although she is supportive of his academic interests outside of work, she worries about his irritability and daytime sleepiness. They go to the appointment together, and she raises her concerns, suggesting that he work on his book an hour a day rather than two. She also suggests that he be "excused" from the normal nighttime family activities a little earlier than usual and that he go back to his previous bedtime. Dr. Song agrees to compromise, and, although the process takes slightly longer than he originally planned, he is proud to publish his book the following year.

Sleep Deprivation

Sleep deprivation can be conceptualized as coming from several sources. Sometimes, sleep loss is a consequence of a conscious choice to stay up late or get up early, often because of external pressures of home or work life. Other times, lack of sleep is due to insomnia or other sleep disorder (e.g., sleep apnea, restless legs syndrome) and may require treatment by a sleep specialist. Hypersomnia and/or insomnia are associated with depression, and lack of restorative sleep is also associated with low and/or irritable mood. Similarly, individuals with anxiety can struggle with sleep initiation (falling asleep) and sleep maintenance (staying asleep). Early morning awakening is common in both mood and anxiety disorders.

Sleep loss due to work demands has received particular attention in the field of medicine. Sleep deprivation can even become a habit during the training years. This deprivation can result because of call responsibilities, excessive workload, or other pressures on trainees to forego sleep. For instance, the encouragement to "always put the patient first" can put pressure on trainees to prioritize clinical services ahead of their own self-care. Once training is complete, the habit of sacrificing self-care can be hard to break. Even though pushing one's own personal limits may be necessary in extreme cases (e.g., to save a life, to handle an emergency), it is not routinely required or advisable because of diminished effectiveness and risk of burnout (Trockel 2019). When a clinician stays up late to catch up on electronic health record documentation or respond to email messages, daytime performance may suffer, and the productivity gained may not be worth the sleep sacrificed.

Sleep deprivation can be detrimental to health in indirect ways as well. For instance, lack of sleep may make it difficult to stick to good eating or exercise habits. Sleep loss can also make it difficult to maintain positive mood. People who are sleep deprived have more difficulty accurately recognizing emotions and reading social cues (Okorie 2019). Evidence that sleep loss increases amygdala response to traumatic images (Krause et al. 2017) is particularly concerning, given the implication that clinicians who have had insufficient sleep may be particularly vulnerable to difficulty coping with trauma they encounter in their work.

Strategies for Optimizing Sleep

Duty hour restrictions (West et al. 2016) have been tried as a strategy for addressing the problems with sleep deprivation among physicians and medical trainees. A wide variety of schedule modifications have been tried with some beneficial effects (Ali et al. 2011; Garland et al. 2012; Panagioti et al. 2017). However, evidence suggests that restricting work hours does not necessarily mean physicians or residents will sleep the recommended amounts (Baldwin et al. 2010). It remains challenging in many settings to balance resident and attending need for sleep with maintaining continuity of patient care and providing ample training opportunities.

In the ever-elusive search for the perfect amount and timing of sleep to optimize function, people have looked to a wide range of tools to help with sleep initiation and maintenance. Medications and behavioral strategies alike have been used with varying levels of success. Sleep medicine experts appear to be in agreement that sleep aids, such as sedative-hypnotics and benzodiazepines, may help with sleep initiation in the short term but do not provide restorative sleep in the long term (Atkin et al. 2018) and are prone to misuse and dependence. In fact, sleep microstructure can be altered such that individuals feel that they have slept but do not get the restorative sleep associated with getting down into deep stage 3 and rapid eye movement (REM) sleep (Manconi et al. 2017). For this reason, most sleep medicine physicians frown on the use of sleep medications, instead favoring a behavioral approach. The same is true for having a drink or two before bed. Alcohol can promote sleep initiation, but it can also interfere with sleep architecture so that sleep is not adequately restorative (Thakkar et al. 2015). Short-term exogenous melatonin use (a naturally occurring hormone produced in the pineal gland and secreted to help regulate circadian rhythms) can be helpful and non–habit forming (Riha 2018).

Ensuring good sleep hygiene is generally the first intervention when working with someone who is struggling to get the proper amount of restorative sleep each night. See Table 11–1 for guidelines.

It is important to try to go to bed and wake up at the same time each day, even on the weekends. Naps during the day should be discouraged because they may make it a challenge to fall asleep at the desired time. People should make sure that their bedroom is an appropriate temperature (not too warm or too cold) and that they reserve the bed for sleep and sex only. When the bed is used for activities, such as doing homework, watching television, or engaging in other relaxation activities and social interaction, the brain and body get confused about the purpose of the bed. The room should be dark and quiet enough to promote sleep. Earplugs and eye masks may be helpful tools. The individual should avoid eating food or drinking large amounts of liquid before bedtime. Stimulating activities, such as showers and use of electronics, should also be avoided. Television, cell phones, e-readers, and computers release shortwave blue light that delays the body's circadian rhythm and suppresses the release of melatonin (Heo et al. 2017). Stimulant medications, including caffeine and nicotine, should be avoided before trying to sleep and can be problematic even hours after their last use. For about an hour before bed, the individual should "wind down" by instituting a relaxing nighttime routine that signals the brain and body that it is time to settle in. Ways to wind down can include drinking herbal tea, taking a bath, reading, working on a puzzle, knitting, and coloring.

If the individual is unable to fall asleep within an hour, it does not make sense to remain in bed. At the same time, it does not help to engage in stimulating activities that will make it even more challenging to fall asleep. Rather than panicking about the loss of sleep and the need to be up in X hours (which is definitely *not* restful), it is generally better to have the individual practice reframing thoughts: "It's OK; I'll just lie here and rest. If nothing else, I will be more relaxed in the morning." He or she can get out of bed and try to read something boring, but now is not the time to pick up the latest thriller or page-turner or download the newest addictive game on a cell phone.

Cognitive-behavioral therapy for insomnia focuses on helping the individual track sleeping and waking patterns and confront beliefs about sleep needs and may involve restricting sleep at certain times (Espie et al.

TABLE 11–1. Sleep hygiene

- Reserve bed for sleeping and sex only.
- Keep naps to less than 30 minutes.
- Exercise daily but avoid stimulating activity right before bedtime.
- Maintain a consistent schedule for bedtime and awakening each morning; try not to vary by more than an hour on weekends or holidays.
- Keep the bedroom dark enough for sleep; use blackout shades or eye masks if needed.
- Make sure that the bedroom is not too hot or too cold and that the bed and bedding are comfortable.
- Avoid heavy meals or drinking a lot of fluids before bedtime.
- Minimize caffeine and nicotine in the afternoon and nighttime hours.
- Avoid alcohol right before bed.
- Minimize use of blue light–emitting electronics before bedtime.
- Practice a consistent bedtime routine of pleasant and calming activities to "wind down."

2019). Rather than fixating on "trying hard to sleep," the focus shifts to "allowing sleep to happen."

Consultation with a sleep medicine specialist is recommended when medical issues may interfere with restorative sleep. Snoring, low or irritable mood, and excessive daytime sleepiness can indicate the presence of sleep apnea, which should be evaluated using a sleep study to determine the appropriate treatment. For example, continuous positive airway pressure (CPAP) can ameliorate symptoms quite efficiently.

Case Example

Gina Brown, a 37-year-old psychiatrist, makes an appointment to see her primary care physician after a scare in which she nodded off at the wheel post call and almost crashed her car. She has been a single parent for 3 years and has recently been going through a period of drama with her ex-husband. He feels that she should increase her alimony and child support payments for their two children and has been threatening to take her to court. Dr. Brown has been taking moonlighting shifts to increase her income for her current alimony payments while also trying to afford the high cost of living in her area. Her worry about the situation has led to significant anxiety, low mood, and trouble sleeping at night. She has been awake until 1:00 or 2:00 each morning contemplating her situation and has difficulty falling asleep. Dr. Brown has experimented with having a glass or two of wine or taking different benzodiazepines or zolpidem to help her fall asleep, but she generally still feels fatigued the following day. She needs to be up each morning when her 4-year-old daughter wakes up, which is typically around 5:30 A.M. Although Dr. Brown is generally able to get out of bed, she finds it challenging to stay awake during the day, especially when driving. Her father has sleep apnea, and she is told that she snores at night, so she asks her primary care physician for a referral to a sleep medicine specialist.

Dr. Brown's situation is complicated by multiple factors. In addition to chronic sleep deprivation secondary to call responsibilities and raising small children, she appears to have a biological vulnerability to sleep apnea, which is well known for causing excessive daytime sleepiness. She is also under tremendous emotional stress and financial pressure that appear to cause mood and anxiety symptoms. People suffering from insomnia often turn to alcohol or sedative-hypnotic medications in the hope of being able to fall asleep earlier. Although these substances can speed sleep initiation, they can disrupt sleep architecture and interfere with the restorative nature of sleep. The daytime sleepiness and tendency to fall asleep at the wheel are particularly concerning because Dr. Brown is the mother of young children and a physician with overnight on-call patient care responsibilities; this underscores the need for urgent evaluation and treatment.

Positive Practices

1. If you feel tempted to stay up late to complete a work task, consider instead choosing sleep as a way of investing in your energy and mental health for the next day. Take note of how this experiment works for you. Many professionals find that chronic sleep deprivation slows down productivity and increases errors to such an extent that it is more efficient to sleep adequately at night and benefit from greater energy for completing important tasks the next day.
2. Mental health conditions, such as anxiety and depression, are known to contribute to challenges with sleep. Often, mood and anxiety are better when sleep is improved, and the converse is true as well: sleep is better when mood and anxiety disorders are adequately treated using a combination of behavioral and medication strategies, including selective serotonin reuptake inhibitors.
3. Alcohol and medications such as sedative-hypnotics and benzodiazepines are generally ineffective in promoting truly restorative sleep. Melatonin, which is naturally released by the pineal gland as a signal to the body to prepare for sleep 8 hours later, can be a useful adjunct to treating insomnia with behavioral strategies.

4. Situations in which a patient is known to snore, has a strong family history of sleep disorders, or has extreme difficulty with excessive daytime sleepiness despite adequate behavioral interventions warrant a consultation with the sleep medicine service. Sleep apnea causes low mood, irritability, and sleepiness and is relatively easily treated using CPAP.

Conclusion

Sleep concerns are common in clinicians because of work, stress, and developmental life stage. Inadequate sleep can lead to problems with physical and mental well-being and can interfere with cognition and good decision-making. Consistent sleep hygiene and specific behavioral changes are typically the most helpful strategies for improving sleep time and quality. Medications for sleep should be used with caution because many compounds can also interfere with sleep quality and architecture. If an individual continues to experience sleep disturbance even after initial attempts to change sleep habits, consultation with a sleep specialist may be warranted. Improvements in the quantity and quality of sleep can greatly affect functioning across domains and can protect patient outcomes.

Exercises
————————o————————

1. **Calculate your sleep time.** Most people need 7–9 hours of sleep each night. Efforts to reduce this amount generally result in daytime sleepiness and challenges regulating the sleep-wake cycle.

   Write your bedtime and wake-up times over the past 5 days below, then calculate how many hours of sleep you received each night. Are you consistently getting at least 7 hours of sleep?

Date	Bedtime	Wake-up time	Hours slept	Sleep quality

2. **Examine your behavior.** Good sleep hygiene and cognitive-behavioral therapy are the first-line interventions for insomnia or difficulties waking up in the morning. Behavioral strategies are by far the most effective in regulating sleep.

   What is the biggest barrier you face to getting adequate sleep?

   _____

   _____

   _____

   On days when you have slept more, what worked?

   _____

   _____

   _____

   If your habit is to stay up too late, try setting a bedtime alarm to remind you how early you need to go to bed in order to get enough restful sleep.

———————O———————

Recommended Resources

Centers for Disease Control and Prevention: Sleep and sleep disorders: resources. Atlanta, GA, Centers for Disease Control and Prevention, 2017. Available at: www.cdc.gov/sleep/resources.html. Accessed July 7, 2019.

Hirshkowitz M, Whiton K, Albert SM, et al: National Sleep Foundation's updated sleep duration recommendations: final report. Sleep Health 1(4):233–243, 2015

Huffington A: The Sleep Revolution: Transforming Your Life, One Night at a Time. New York, Harmony, 2016

National Sleep Foundation: Healthy sleep tips. Arlington, VA, National Sleep Foundation, 2019. Available at: www.sleepfoundation.org/articles/healthy-sleep-tips. Accessed July 7, 2019.

Noordsy DL (ed): Lifestyle Psychiatry. Washington, DC, American Psychiatric Association Publishing, 2019

References

Ali NA, Hammersley J, Hoffmann SP, et al: Continuity of care in intensive care units: a cluster-randomized trial of intensivist staffing. Am J Respir Crit Care Med 184(7):803–808, 2011 21719756

Atkin T, Comai S, Gobbi G: Drugs for insomnia beyond benzodiazepines: pharmacology, clinical applications, and discovery. Pharmacol Rev 70(2):197–245, 2018 29487083

Baldwin DC Jr, Daugherty SR, Ryan P, Yaghmour NA: Changes in resident work and sleep hours 1999 to 2009: results from a survey of 4 specialties. J Grad Med Educ 2(4):656–658, 2010 22132295

Boardman JM, Bei B, Mellor A, et al: The ability to self-monitor cognitive performance during 60 h total sleep deprivation and following 2 nights recovery sleep. J Sleep Res 27(4):e12633, 2018 29159907

Espie CA, Emsley R, Kyle SD, et al: Effect of digital cognitive behavioral therapy for insomnia on health, psychological well-being, and sleep-related quality of life: a randomized clinical trial. JAMA Psychiatry. 76(1):21–30, 2019 30264137

Ferrie JE, Shipley MJ, Cappuccio FP, et al: A prospective study of change in sleep duration: associations with mortality in the Whitehall II cohort. Sleep 30(12):1659–1666, 2007 18246975

Garland A, Roberts D, Graff L: Twenty-four-hour intensivist presence: a pilot study of effects on intensive care unit patients, families, doctors, and nurses. Am J Respir Crit Care Med 185(7):738–743, 2012 22246176

Harrison Y, Horne JA: The impact of sleep deprivation on decision making: a review. J Exp Psychol Appl 6(3):236–249, 2000 11014055

Heo JY, Kim K, Fava M, et al: Effects of smartphone use with and without blue light at night in healthy adults: a randomized, double-blind, cross-over, placebo-controlled comparison. J Psychiatr Res 87:61–70, 2017 28017916

Hirshkowitz M, Whiton K, Albert SM, et al: National Sleep Foundation's updated sleep duration recommendations: final report. Sleep Health 1(4):233–243, 2015 29073398

Krause AJ, Simon EB, Mander BA, et al: The sleep-deprived human brain. Nat Rev Neurosci 18(7):404–418, 2017 28515433

Liu Y, Wheaton AG, Chapman DP, et al: Prevalence of healthy sleep duration among adults—United States, 2014. MMWR Morb Mortal Wkly Rep 65(6):137–141, 2016 26890214

Maier JG, Nissen C: Sleep and memory: mechanisms and implications for psychiatry. Curr Opin Psychiatry 30(6):480–484, 2017 28858009

Manconi M, Ferri R, Miano S, et al: Sleep architecture in insomniacs with severe benzodiazepine abuse. Clin Neurophysiol 28(6):875–881, 2017 28399441

Okorie CU: Sleep, in The Art and Science of Physician Wellbeing: A Handbook for Physicians and Trainees. Edited by Roberts LW, Trockel MT. Cham, Switzerland, Springer, 2019, pp 255–278

Olson EJ, Drage LA, Auger RR: Sleep deprivation, physician performance, and patient safety. Chest 136(5):1389–1396, 2009 19892678

Panagioti M, Panagopoulou E, Bower P, et al: Controlled interventions to reduce burnout in physicians: a systematic review and meta-analysis. JAMA Intern Med 177(2):195–205, 2017 27918798

Rechtschaffen A, Bergmann BM: Sleep deprivation in the rat by the disk-over-water method. Behav Brain Res 69(1–2):55–63, 1995 7546318

Riha RL: The use and misuse of exogenous melatonin in the treatment of sleep disorders. Curr Opin Pulm Med 24(6):543–548, 2018 30148726

Rothschild JM, Keohane CA, Rogers S, et al: Risks of complications by attending physicians after performing nighttime procedures. JAMA 302(14):1565–1572, 2009 19826026

Tamakoshi A, Ohno Y, JACC Study Group: Self-reported sleep duration as a predictor of all-cause mortality: results from the JACC study, Japan. Sleep 27(1):51–54, 2004 14998237

Thakkar MM, Sharma R, Sahota P: Alcohol disrupts sleep homeostasis. Alcohol 49(4):299–310, 2015 25499829

Trockel MT: Calling, compassionate self, and cultural norms in medicine, in The Art and Science of Physician Wellbeing: A Handbook for Physicians and Trainees. Edited by Roberts LW, Trockel MT. Cham, Switzerland, Springer, 2019, pp 3–17

West CP, Dyrbye LN, Erwin PJ, Shanafelt TD: Interventions to prevent and reduce physician burnout: a systematic review and meta-analysis. Lancet 388(10057):2272–2281, 2016 27692469

ॐ

CHAPTER 12

Relationships and Social Connection

Social relationships subtly embrace us in the warmth of self-affirmation, the whispers of encouragement, and the meaningfulness of belonging. They are fundamental to our emotional fulfillment, behavioral adjustment, and cognitive function.

Hughes et al. 2004

Humans are a social species, naturally seeking reliably secure and safe social connections throughout their life span. Mental health professionals, however, often find themselves in isolated circumstances, despite the fact that the very nature of their work involves being around and caring for others. They immerse themselves in the emotional lives of their patients and their patients' families and work to address others' loneliness while sometimes neglecting their own.

Schedules for psychiatrists and psychologists can become fully booked with back-to-back patient appointments, teaching, supervision, research, and administrative responsibilities. Although some of these responsibilities involve interaction with other professionals, there may not be time or space for meaningful interpersonal interactions or the informal chatting that increases a sense of belonging and camaraderie in the workplace. Even the architectural design of clinical buildings and research laboratories may inadvertently lead to isolative tendencies as colleagues work alone in their offices behind closed doors.

Mental health care professionals are urged to develop and maintain meaningful social connections. Purposefully and consistently devoting energy to this endeavor can decrease loneliness and social disconnection,

231

both of which are notably risky for general physical health and psychological well-being. Purposeful social engagement lays the foundation for numerous long-lasting, positive effects. These effects include lifetime friendships, professional fulfillment, collaborations, opportunities for mentorship, discovery of new interests, and development of social networks to mitigate the loneliness that sometimes accompanies retirement and aging.

Lack of Social Connectivity and Loneliness

Loneliness can be thought of as a disconnect between what an individual expects and wants from a particular relationship and what the individual is actually receiving from that relationship, resulting in dissonance. It follows, then, that loneliness can be experienced even when one is physically near other people (e.g., at home, at work, in public) because it is the consequence of perceived differentials in expectations.

According to a meta-analysis of more than 177,000 participants, personal and friendship networks have shrunk over the last 35 years (Wrzus et al. 2013). Prevalence rates of loneliness in the general population can range from 10% to 30% (Beutel et al. 2017). A study of psychologists found that about 10% endorsed distress from loneliness (Thoreson et al. 1989). Interestingly, a longitudinal study of 4,000 American workers found that individuals with graduate degrees endorse more loneliness than those whose highest degrees were an undergraduate or high school degree (Achor et al. 2018). In fact, individuals with law and medical degrees reported the greatest degree of loneliness, approximately 20% more than individuals with a Ph.D.

Consequences of the Lack of Social Connectivity and Loneliness

The literature on loneliness is clear: it is detrimental to physical and psychological health. Loneliness is associated with various physical health manifestations, such as increased inflammation and cardiovascular disease, and has been shown to increase the odds of premature mortality by 14%–19%, even when adjusting for demographic factors and baseline health (Holwerda et al. 2016; Wrzus et al. 2013). A meta-analysis of 148 studies, including more than 300,000 people, found that study participants with stronger social relationships had a significantly higher likelihood of surviving over the course of the studies compared with individuals with weaker social relationships (Holt-Lunstad et al. 2010). Specifically, the degree of difference was comparable to double that of the impact of obesity and roughly equivalent to smoking 15 cigarettes daily. Individuals with higher levels of loneliness tend to visit their physicians more frequently (Beutel et al. 2017).

Psychological consequences of loneliness also cannot be ignored. Loneliness can increase irritability and other symptoms of depression as well as reduce sleep. An additional risk associated with social disconnection and loneliness is that they can become self-fulfilling prophecies. An individual may lose confidence in his or her social support system, reduce engagement with said system, and then become relatively more detached.

Loneliness also impacts workplace engagement. For example, research participants who reported higher degrees of loneliness also reported fewer promotions, lower job satisfaction, and a higher likelihood of quitting their jobs within 6 months (Achor et al. 2018). Thus, loneliness can have a substantial economic impact. Among medical residents, several studies have demonstrated a link between feelings of loneliness and burnout (Rogers et al. 2016; Shapiro et al. 2015). A brief, three-item assessment of loneliness (Table 12–1) is useful to identify this association (Hughes et al. 2004).

Finally, loneliness and other aspects of social disconnectedness (i.e., living alone, loss of a spouse, lack of social support, social isolation) are important risk factors for suicide, particularly among older adults (Van Orden and Conwell 2011). These findings are consistent with the interpersonal theory of suicide (Figure 12–1), which hypothesizes that two factors—thwarted belongingness and a feeling of being a burden—are associated with suicide, particularly in older adults (Van Orden et al. 2010). Thwarted belongingness refers not only to social connections but also to the quality of those connections: "Thwarted belongingness is a painful mental state that results from an unmet need to belong—a need to feel connected to others in a positive and caring way" (Van Orden and Conwell 2011, p. 6). Therefore, fostering an awareness of the need to feel connected in *positive and caring ways*—essentially, to belong—and finding ways to meet this need are crucial to preventing suicide in mental health professionals.

Benefits of Strong Social Connections

The potential beneficial outcomes of strong social relationships are compelling. Research has demonstrated that these connections may

---

TABLE 12–1. Three-item loneliness scale

The following questions are about how you feel about different aspects of your
   life. For each one, tell me how often you feel that way.
1.   First, how often do you feel that you lack companionship: hardly ever,
     some of the time, or often?
2.   How often do you feel left out: hardly ever, some of the time, or often?
3.   How often do you feel isolated from others? (Is it hardly ever, some of the
     time, or often?)

Scoring: 1 = "hardly ever"; 2 = "some of the time"; 3 = "often."
Total score = sum of item scores. Higher scores indicate greater loneliness.

Source.   Adapted from Hughes ME, Waite LJ, Hawkley LC, Cacioppo JT: A short
scale for measuring loneliness in large surveys: results from two population-based
studies. *Research on Aging* 26(6):655–672, 2004. © 2004 by SAGE Publications. Reprinted by permission of SAGE Publications, Inc.

---

have a wide variety of impacts, such as extending longevity and reducing
the risk of psychological disturbances (Figure 12–2).

Intervention research that addressed loneliness in older adults has
demonstrated that even relatively straightforward interventions that
seek to connect older adults to others (e.g., telephone outreach, increasing engagement in volunteer and peer support activities) can reduce the
risk of suicide (Van Orden and Conwell 2011). The following vignette
provides an example of one clinician's changing experience of loneliness
across her professional life and the ways in which increasing connection
with colleagues and trainees in her later years improved her sense of
well-being.

Vignette

After completing her residency, Smita Tal spent 5 years providing therapy and medication evaluations in the clinic where she trained. She then
left the clinic and entered private practice, where her years of training,
empathetic and skilled approach, and reputation as an outstanding psychiatrist allowed her to build and sustain a thriving practice. She enjoyed
the flexible hours her independent practice afforded her, especially as she
and her partner raised their children. She attended a weekly consultation
session for 15 years and was pleased with the level of comfort and connectivity she felt with colleagues. After her youngest child left home for
college, she began to wonder about having deeper, more meaningful relationships, both within and outside of her field of work. She realized how
much she missed mentorship. She had not truly received nor provided it

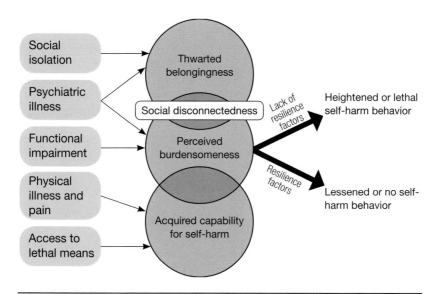

FIGURE 12–1. Interpersonal theory of suicide.

The five boxes on the left of the figure represent key risk factors for lethal self-harm, as derived from psychological autopsy studies. The three circles in the middle of the figure represent the three key constructs posited to lead to lethal self-harm. The arrows connecting the risk factors (boxes) and the three key constructs (circles) represent hypothesized psychological mechanisms.
Source. Adapted from Van Orden and Conwell 2011.

since she left training. She also reflected that 20 years of being a hardworking, full-time psychiatrist, mother, and wife meant she had not invested in deepening her friendships outside of the office as much as she wished she had. Dr. Tal felt the heavy throb of loneliness and a growing sense of dread about returning to the office. This monotony plagued her for some time. She was vulnerable and honest about these feelings with her consultation group. They showed immediate support of her and encouraged her to seek deeper, meaningful relationships and connections. They also noted and empathized with the normality of feeling the heavy emptiness of her home after both of her adult children moved away. The consultation group also asked about the function of her loneliness. In response, Dr. Tal reflected that she felt it meant she needed to seek connections. She decided to reach out to various community clinics to apply for teaching, mentorship, and supervisory roles. The clinics enthusiastically welcomed her interest, and she had interviews set up within a month. She also reached out to local community acquaintances who were parents of her children's friends and offered to host a meet-up for empty nesters. Dr. Tal felt more esteem and less disconnection after putting these actions into motion.

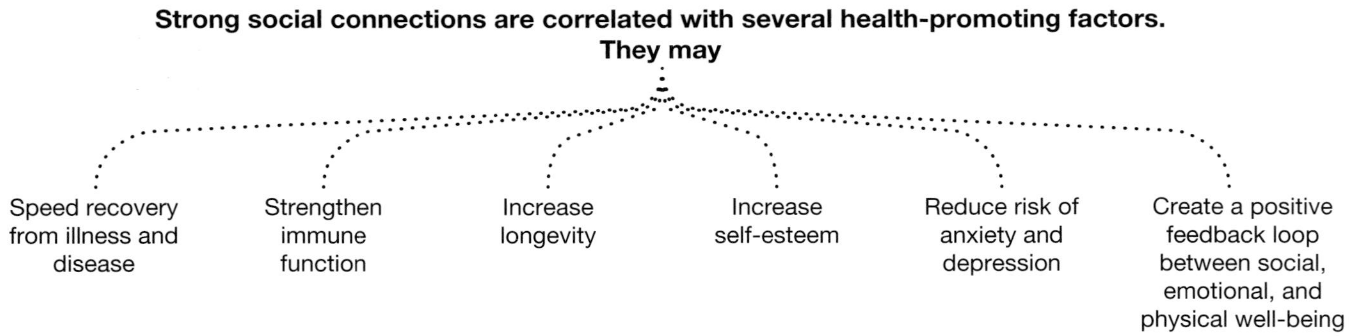

Strong social connections are correlated with several health-promoting factors. They may

Speed recovery from illness and disease

Strengthen immune function

Increase longevity

Increase self-esteem

Reduce risk of anxiety and depression

Create a positive feedback loop between social, emotional, and physical well-being

FIGURE 12–2. Correlates of strong social connections.

Source. Image created by Athena Robinson.

Creating Opportunity for Connectedness

Social disconnection and feelings of loneliness can be experienced at any life stage for mental health clinicians, whether in private practice or specialty clinics, in teaching and research roles, or as trainees. Because no one is immune to the ups and downs of social connectivity and accompanying feelings of loneliness, it is important to think proactively about how to stay engaged socially in the multiple environments of one's life: work, home, community, etc. After all, the function of the emotion of loneliness itself may signal the need to feel connected to others and may propel an individual in that direction.

Case Example

Dr. Andrew Schwartz is a 72-year-old psychologist who has run his own private practice for more than 30 years. He continues to enjoy his practice and feels he has helped many patients. He and his wife, Karen, who retired from teaching 3 years ago, have raised three children, are financially secure (although he worries about whether they may outlive their savings), and feel as though they have a happy, stable marriage. He works approximately 30 hours per week, and he exercises alone at the gym 2–3 days per week. Although he was raised in an observant Jewish household and identifies as Jewish, he and his wife do not belong to a synagogue and are not involved in community or civic organizations. They have a small group of three other couples they see occasionally for dinner. These arrangements are always made by Karen and the other women. The husbands join in but do not see one another socially except when their wives make plans. In the last 2 years, since turning 70, Dr. Schwartz has noticed increased feelings of loneliness, even when he is with his wife. Although he enjoys gathering socially with their friends, he realizes they have not made any new friends in years and wonders if this is normal. Part of him would like to cut back on his work and spend time on hobbies he used to enjoy, such as woodworking, but he is worried that this solitary activity will not curb his loneliness. He is also hesitant about whether he still has the manual dexterity he once had for the precision of woodworking. He has never volunteered before but has often encouraged patients to do so, believing volunteer work can help them find meaning, meet other people, or add structure to their days.

Despite being aware of his loneliness, he refrains from discussing it with his wife because he is concerned it would hurt her feelings. He has not shared his innermost thoughts with anyone because he has few close friends. He also feels a sense of shame that, as a psychologist, he has not figured out on his own how to address these personal issues. Thinking about what he might suggest to a patient in his own situation, Dr. Schwartz wonders about taking a woodworking class, volunteering, or joining a synagogue. These ideas percolate, but as time goes by, he fails to act on them. Dr. Schwartz feels ashamed and "stuck," while experiencing a lack of meaning in his own work. He ponders if he is depressed. Gradually, he drops his time at the gym and spends more time lying in bed during mornings when he does not have patients scheduled. He has thoughts of wondering if "it is all worth it," although he has not formulated any specific actions to end his life.

Dr. Schwartz's situation is far from unique, whether among middle-age and older adults in general or aging mental health professionals more specifically. Dr. Schwartz's case, as initially described, is relatively mild, in the sense that he has a number of protective factors that—if optimized—could help him prevent increased loneliness. A number of concerning issues are illustrated. Although mental health professionals are trained to recognize and discuss feelings, the assumption that they will be able to access adequate support from family and friends is not necessarily warranted. Psychiatrists and psychologists are human, too, and can become "stuck" in their own maladaptive patterns. As illustrated by Dr. Schwartz's case, feelings of shame are extremely common and can prevent psychiatrists and psychologists from addressing their own needs.

As time goes by, Dr. Schwartz's loneliness begins to morph into depression. He may be at risk for a number of negative outcomes, including declining mental and physical health and even suicide. If the scenario changed slightly by identifying Dr. Schwartz as a widower with few friends, his risk would increase significantly. Older men, particularly those who are socially isolated, are at heightened risk of suicide. As predicted by the interpersonal theory of suicide, a sense of thwarted belongingness is one of the key predictors of suicide in older adults.

Optimizing positive factors for Dr. Schwartz include joining a synagogue or identifying other ways to explore his spirituality with others, finding ways to volunteer in a social setting, taking an exercise class (or even walking with friends), or signing up for a fun and relaxing woodworking class. His concerns about woodworking as a solitary activity are appropriate. Although having hobbies can be beneficial, activities that address the need for belonging and connection may be more relevant in cases such as Dr. Schwartz's.

Positive Practices

1. Avoid pathologizing loneliness. It is a universal and an expected human experience, not a feeling to be ashamed of. Retreating into loneliness can cause social disconnection over time.

2. Address maladaptive cognitions. Be mindful of your own thoughts and whether or not your interpretations of loneliness are accurate. Avoid creating a self-fulfilling prophecy. A meta-analysis revealed that interventions have demonstrated successful reductions in loneliness by having individuals address and challenge their own negative thoughts about loneliness (Masi et al. 2011).

3. Leverage the experience of loneliness to inspire ways to connect with others rather than retreat into shame or depression. The very emotion of loneliness can be a beautiful (yes, beautiful!) signal that you truly do desire and seek to deepen relationships.

4. Try new things. Sign up for a recreational team or league, game night, book club, or improv or meet-up event. Self-motivation may require addressing the self-talk individuals may engage in (e.g., "I won't like anyone there," "I'm not a joiner"). Try using open and compassionate self-talk to encourage yourself. Trying out a new activity or group does not imply a lifetime commitment.

5. Be yourself. You do not need to change who you are or force a connection if there does not appear to be a match. Practice the self-acceptance you would encourage in your patients.

6. Connect with colleagues and friends. Connecting online as well as in person can help you stay in touch easily. Log on to LinkedIn and read about your colleagues' latest publications or press releases. Join webinars about a topic you are eager to learn more about. Volunteer to write a blog post and welcome collegial feedback. On the other hand, if you notice that spending time online affects your mood negatively, identify what emotions are being activated (e.g., some individuals tend to engage in negative self-talk and social comparison when they read about others' accomplishments). Spending time online can be a double-edged sword, and it is important to find ways that an online presence works for you, while avoiding the trap of replacing in-person relationships with virtual ones.

7. Practice thoughtful disclosure. Research demonstrates that iteratively increasing the depth of questions and answers between strangers can spawn friendships in short bouts of time (Aron et al. 1997). Ask about small things ("How do you commute to work?") at first and then build up to the relevant disclosure factor associated with your questions ("It's been challenging for me to find a consultation group I truly connect with. How did you do it?").

8. Volunteer. Within or outside of your workplace, volunteering for a cause that is meaningful to you can inspire new opportunities to

connect with people with whom you already have something in common.

9. Consider group engagement. Engagement or reengagement, even on a small level, with a spiritual, religious, cultural, political, or other community-based organization may be one way to connect with others.

10. Find a shared sense of meaning with your colleagues. Identifying a collective mission among colleagues can foster a sense of unity and drive workplace initiatives.

Conclusion

The widely felt, and empirically documented, rising tide of decreased social connectivity impacts psychiatrists and psychologists as well as the general public. Because of their intense, long, and often challenging professional activities, mental health professionals are at risk for experiencing social disconnection, loneliness, and isolation. Social disconnection has important negative effects on emotional and physical health, increases risk for burnout, and contributes to suicide risk.

Self-reflection on one's degree of social connectedness and loneliness and thoughtful action planning on how to increase and deepen relationships are important self-care behaviors for mental health professionals across the span of their careers and beyond. The dividends paid for investing in social connections and relationships are well worth the investment of time and effort. Furthermore, modeling ways of building new social connections and deepening existing ones sends an important signal to families, patients, friends, peers, junior colleagues, and trainees that taking care of oneself in this essential human way is vital to well-being.

Exercises

──────○──────

1. **Reflect on current levels of connectivity.** The practice of openly and nonjudgmentally reflecting on your own degree of social connectedness and loneliness can illuminate opportunity for change. It also presents a chance to debunk shame around feelings of isolation in your personal or professional life. Openly ask yourself the following questions:

How satisfied are you with your current degree of social connectedness?

Do you think your mental health could benefit from creating new or deepening current relationships?

Could you benefit from social skills strengthening? Social skills are just like any other skill. They take development and practice. Be honest and nonjudgmental with yourself if you need to bolster your social skills. For example, do you know how to comfortably strike up a conversation with a stranger or acquaintance? Do you feel confident in turning an acquaintance into a friendship?

2. **Craft daily moments of connection.** Improving social connectedness requires purposeful and repetitive action. Make a small daily or weekly effort to invest in and nurture relationships (e.g., send a text or email message, invite someone out to lunch or for a walk, join the lunchtime yoga group in your office). Where could you actively seek additional relationships, in and out of the office?

---

3. **Build and maintain relationships.** Build relationships with individuals you admire in your department, whether or not they are immediately within your area of expertise. Write at least two actions you will take this week to strengthen these connections.

―――――――――○―――――――――

Recommended Resources

Barres B: The Autobiography of a Transgender Scientist. Cambridge, MA, MIT Press, 2018

Baumeister RF, Leary MR: The need to belong: desire for interpersonal attachments as a fundamental human motivation. Psychol Bull 117(3):497–529, 1995

Gottman J: Making relationships work: part 1 (video). Seattle, WA, Gottman Institute, November 30, 2009. Available at: www.youtube.com/watch?v=LLXX8wzvT7c. Accessed June 7, 2019.

Gottman J: The Art of Relationships (podcast audio). September 21, 2016. Available at: www.stitcher.com/podcast/biola-university/the-art-of-relationships-podcast. Accessed June 7, 2019.

Gottman J, et al: The Gottman relationship blog. Seattle, WA, Gottman Institute, 2019. Available at: www.gottman.com/blog. Accessed June 7, 2019.

Noordsy DL (ed): Lifestyle Psychiatry. Washington, DC, American Psychiatric Association Publishing, 2019

Perel E: The Arc of Love (podcast audio). 2018. Available at: www.estherperel.com/podcast. Accessed May 20, 2019.

Yalom ID: Becoming Myself: A Psychiatrist's Memoir. London, Hachette, 2017

References

Achor S, Kellerman GR, Reece A, Robichaux A: America's loneliest workers, according to research. Harvard Business Review, March 19, 2018. Available at: https://hbr.org/2018/03/americas-loneliest-workers-according-to-research. Accessed May 20, 2019

Aron A, Melinat E, Aron EN, et al: The experimental generation of interpersonal closeness: a procedure and some preliminary findings. Personality and Social Psychology Bulletin 23(4):363–377, 1997

Beutel ME, Klein EM, Brähler E, et al: Loneliness in the general population: prevalence, determinants and relations to mental health. BMC Psychiatry 17(1):97, 2017 28320380

Holt-Lunstad J, Smith TB, Layton B: Social relationships and mortality risk: a meta-analytic review. PLoS Med 7(7):e1000316, 2010 20668659

Holwerda TJ, van Tilburg TG, Deeg DJH, et al: Impact of loneliness and depression on mortality: results from the Longitudinal Ageing Study Amsterdam. Br J Psychiatry 209(2):127–134, 2016 27103680

Hughes ME, Waite LJ, Hawkley LC, Cacioppo JT: A short scale for measuring loneliness in large surveys: results from two population-based studies. Res Aging 26(6):655–672, 2004 18504506

Masi CM, Chen HY, Hawkley LC, Cacioppo JT: A meta-analysis of interventions to reduce loneliness. Pers Soc Psychol Rev 5(3):219–266, 2011 20716644

Rogers E, Polonijo AN, Carpiano RM: Getting by with a little help from friends and colleagues: testing how residents' social support networks affect loneliness and burnout. Can Fam Physician 62(11):e677–e683, 2016

Shapiro J, Zhang B, Warm EJ: Residency as a social network: burnout, loneliness, and social network centrality. J Grad Med Educ 7(4):617–623, 2015 26692975

Thoreson RW, Miller M, Krauskopf CJ: The distressed psychologist: prevalence and treatment considerations. Prof Psychol Res Pr 20(3):153–158, 1989

Van Orden K, Conwell Y: Suicides in late life. Curr Psychiatry Rep 13(3):234–241, 2011 21369952

Van Orden KA, Witte TK, Cukrowicz KC, et al: The interpersonal theory of suicide. Psychol Rev 117(2):575–600, 2010 20438238

Wrzus C, Hänel M, Wagner J, Neyer FJ: Social network changes and life events across the life span: a meta-analysis. Psychol Bull 139(1):53–80, 2013 22642230

CHAPTER 13

Psychiatric Care and Psychotherapy

Even our misfortunes are part of our belongings.

Antoine de Saint-Exupéry

Mental health professionals as a group have an uneasy relationship to their own mental health treatment, particularly during training years. When it comes to their patients, psychiatrists and psychologists tend to speak of counseling and pharmacotherapy from a place of nonjudgment, designating treatments as self-care practices that promote wellness, self-awareness, and ongoing growth and learning. They readily assure reluctant patients that therapy is not synonymous with pathology, failure, or brokenness but, in fact, is a sign of openness, resilience, and self-esteem. However, as professionals in the field, psychiatrists and psychologists too often fail to provide colleagues, trainees, or even themselves the same compassion or transparency.

Roughly three-quarters of mental health professionals will seek therapeutic treatment at some point in their career (Norcross 2005), and the vast majority (>90%) will proclaim it useful both personally and professionally. Outside of a few urban communities where therapy is more openly discussed, the belief widely persists that seasoned professionals do not need therapy. Understanding the numerous benefits of seeking care, the historical barriers to access and openness, and the array of services available to support mental health professionals may help clinicians embrace personal practices to enhance well-being.

Barriers to Care

As described in Chapter 4, "Approaches to Mental Health Care for Fellow Clinicians," concerns about confidentiality and stigma top the list for reasons psychiatrists and psychologists are reticent to seek mental health treatment, even when they are struggling with work-related burnout, depression, or vicarious trauma (Barnett et al. 2007; Moutier et al. 2009). Studies suggest that the majority of physicians experience embarrassment at seeking treatment (Brimstone et al. 2007), and roughly a quarter endorse treating their own chronic medical conditions rather than entering professional care. These concerns are particularly acute for trainees, occurring at every stage of development (undergraduates, medical students, residents, interns, postdoctoral fellows) and across the mental health disciplines (e.g., psychology, psychiatry, counseling, nursing).

Trainees report fears that seeking treatment will result in their being found unfit to practice professionally (Baker and Sen 2016). As a result, they tend to endorse a preference for peer or nonprofessional consultation. For instance, surveyed medical and psychology trainees responded to vignettes by endorsing greater likelihood of talking to a family member or friend than a professional for a mental health concern. Only a quarter of surveyed undergraduate psychology students anticipated that they would seek treatment for symptomatic stress, anxiety, or depression (Thomas et al. 2014). Trainees also reported being less likely to talk openly about difficult cases with attendings than with peers out of concern that their evaluations would be negatively impacted or they would appear unstable (Houpy et al. 2017).

Concerns that seeking treatment casts doubt on a mental health professional's competence reflect a historical culture in which doctors were viewed as superhuman. Common humanity, the essential universal humanness of all people, was deemphasized for physicians. Rather, physicians report being steeped in messaging that the competent professional is invulnerable, "possessing a supernatural resilience" (Baker and Sen 2016). This contrasts sharply with the reality that most seasoned clinicians use therapy services (Norcross 2005) and points to a need to shift the culture of how psychiatrists and psychologists talk as a profession about use of services. As third-wave therapies emphasizing self-compassion, acceptance, and mindfulness come to light (see Chapter 9, "Mindfulness and Spiritual Well-Being"), the time is right for supporting a change: viewing physicians for what they are first and foremost—people with all of the passions, needs, and concerns of any other human being.

Mental health professionals seeking treatment worry about confidentiality and dual relationships. A study of medical and psychology students indicated that both groups report confidentiality concerns for mental but not physical health treatment (Brimstone et al. 2007). Residents report greater concerns over their alcohol abuse and panic attacks being made public than about diabetes or hypertension (Moutier et al. 2009). Further exacerbating confidentiality issues, psychiatrists and psychologists seeking care may have difficulty finding a treating clinician with whom they or their close colleagues do not already have an existing professional relationship because therapy circles are often overlapping (Barnett et al. 2007). Clinicians who are experienced at treating other mental health professionals are a more limited group. These barriers have not prevented most seasoned clinicians from seeking care, but they suggest the need to better support trainees who appear most vulnerable to stigma.

Benefits of Mental Health Professionals Seeking Care

Despite the complexities, professional consultation or therapy can be essential to self-care. When mental health professionals engage in their own personal psychotherapy, both the clinician and the clinician's patients benefit. Numerous authors report that individual or group supervision, psychotherapy, peer support, and colleague assistance programs result in great benefit to mental health professionals who use them (e.g., Barnett and Hillard 2001; Mahoney 1997; Norcross 2005). In fact, surveys of more than 4,000 therapist-patients find that the vast majority (88%–90% or more) report treatment to have been personally helpful (Orlinsky et al. 2005; Orlinsky and Rønnestad 2005), and 94% report that the experience was additionally helpful to career development. Mental health professionals value experiential learning through therapy, supervision, and practicum field placements over didactic courses and workshop learning (Norcross 2005). Experienced health professionals acknowledge the benefits of supervision and peer support across their careers (Barnett et al. 2007).

There are also gains to patients, although not necessarily via anticipated mechanisms. Research to date has found no evidence that therapists' participation in personal therapy improves outcomes for their own patients (although studies are criticized for small samples and lack of a control group). Process-experiential elements are correlated, with patients rating greater warmth, empathy, genuineness, countertransference management, and relational emphasis for mental health professionals who have themselves undergone therapy (Norcross 2005).

Selecting a Therapist

The goals of physician-patients shift over the life span, with most experienced mental health professionals reporting that they have sought therapy more than once and for different reasons at various life phases (Norcross 2005). Psychiatrists and psychologists also do not necessarily seek treatment from within their own theoretical approach, with more individuals seeking insight-oriented versus behavioral treatment, regardless of their theoretical orientation. Psychoanalytic, psychodynamic, and humanistic professionals are the most likely to seek orientation-congruent therapy, whereas cognitive-behavioral therapists seek like treatment 60% of the time and behaviorists seek a strict behavioral intervention less than 10% of the time (Norcross 2005). A like-minded professional offers a familiar approach with a shared values system, which promotes validation, modeling, and solidification of theoretical identity (Norcross 2005). On the other hand, seeking therapy with a psychiatrist or psychologist from a different orientation offers flexibility and the opportunity to expand one's experience and gain an appreciation for the myriad effective ways of working therapeutically. Seeking a mental health professional outside of one's preferred orientation is also in keeping with studies finding that the most seasoned and skilled psychotherapists draw from multiple orientations and approaches rather than adhering strictly to a single protocol (Norcross 2005).

The preferred demographics of treating clinicians have also changed over time, reflecting changes in the field. Preferred clinician gender shifted from male to an equal balance of male and female; younger-generation patients shifted from psychiatrists to psychologists for treatment (Norcross 2005). Following this trend, it is anticipated that as access concerns propel the increase of employment of master's-level clinicians, therapist-patients may increasingly seek care from clinical social workers, marital and family therapists, and nurse practitioners. The best therapist fit is, of course, personal and should match the clinical and process-experiential needs of the clinician-patient. Nevertheless, there are commonalities across studies as to what mental health practitioners endorse seeking when they look for a therapist. These qualities include experience, competence, and reputation for excellence or for being a "therapist's therapist," as well as a style that is warm and caring and active and involved (Norcross 2005). Clinician-patients also emphasize the importance of selecting a professional outside of their usual network to reduce concern over dual relationships (Baker and Sen 2016).

Valuable Alternatives to Therapy

In the last 20 years, personal practices that help mental health professionals enhance their personal as well as professional development have expanded from psychotherapy into self-directed mindfulness and meditation-based programs and self-practice/self-reflection programs (Bennett-Levy and Finlay-Jones 2018). Mindfulness-based cognitive therapy, mindfulness-based stress reduction, and self-compassion/loving-kindness practices offer new avenues for experiential learning and mindfulness, as discussed in Chapter 9. Equally valuable in the clinician's self-care arsenal are ongoing supervision, consultation, and both professional and peer-to-peer coaching and mentorship. Consultation can take a wide range of forms. See Table 13–1 for suggestions.

The following vignette illustrates how one clinician overcame his initial reservations and explored a consultation group to access additional peer supervision and support from colleagues.

Vignette

Julio Marin is a marriage and family therapist in his fourth year of running a private practice. With a thriving business and full caseload, he easily fills his days with patient appointments. Despite his full days, he increasingly finds himself feeling isolated. Although he initially enjoyed the absence of meetings and required trainings that were prevalent in his agency work, he now finds he misses scheduled face-to-face time with colleagues, the camaraderie of agency life, and the ability to pop into a coworker's office between patients to run a scenario by him or her or to share a moment of support over a particularly tough session. He has a full social life, yet his workdays feel long and surprisingly lonely.

After a particularly challenging week, Dr. Marin shares his experience over lunch with a former coworker, Lillian Taira, who suggests that he consider a peer consultation group. He expresses initial reservations and concern about giving up a billable hour, about whether he really "needs" consultation, and about how he would even find the right group. Further conversation with Dr. Taira reminds him that the weekly hour is an investment in himself and his practice. He recalls that he has always enjoyed supervision, both to learn new approaches and to hone his technique, and also for the opportunity to connect with others and feel understood in his work. Dr. Taira shares her experience of creating a consultation group by asking like-minded peers to come together. She acknowledges that the group she joined initially had not been the right

TABLE 13–1. Finding or creating the right consultation for your needs

	Considerations and questions to ask yourself
Frequency	Whether professional or peer to peer, consultation can be ongoing or a one-time event. The following factors may help inform a decision about frequency of consultation:
	• Do you have a unique question (e.g., an ethical dilemma, a legal issue, a recent sticky session)?
	• Are you looking for ongoing support (e.g., goal of lifelong professional growth)?
	• Do you desire to learn a new approach?
	• Have you experienced recent substantive changes (e.g., starting private practice, shifting to a new patient population, struggling with a challenging case)?
Expertise	Paid consultants can be particularly useful in the following situations:
	• Learning a new treatment or technique
	• Enhancing a specific skill
	• Learning a new business practice
	Respected colleagues often can be equally beneficial and more cost-effective for consultation in the following situations:
	• To check your thinking
	• To get multiple perspectives
	• To stay current with the literature
	• To keep adherent to treatment approaches
	• To receive ongoing validation and support
Content	Identify your desired area of growth for effective ongoing consultation and select an expert in this area or like-minded advanced peers:
	• A particular treatment approach (e.g., CBT, ACT)
	• A particular specialty area (e.g., eating disorders, trauma)
	• Other themes (e.g., building a private practice)
Participants	Consultation group membership can have various forms.
	• Membership may be open or closed.
	• The group may comprise people who work together or who know each other through less regular contact (e.g., conferences), or members may be unknown to one another prior to joining.

TABLE 13–1. Finding or creating the right consultation for your needs *(continued)*

Considerations and questions to ask yourself

| Setting | • The group may form first and then hire an expert consultant, or individuals may be brought together by a consultant whom multiple people have sought out.
Consider the pros and cons of joining an existing group (ease) versus building one (tailored fit).
Consider whether the group will meet in person or remotely, capitalizing on telecommunication.
• In-person meetings enhance intimacy of support.
• Remote meetings may be practically realistic for accessing an expert or group of like-minded individuals who do not live in proximity to one another or to cut costs of time away from a clinical practice. |

Note. ACT=acceptance and commitment therapy; CBT=cognitive-behavioral therapy.

fit, but by proactively approaching others in her area of specialty whose work she respected, she was able to gather a small group of early-career clinicians in private practice. They collectively hired a consultant, and the group has gone on to meet consistently for many years, even changing consultants periodically to allow them to learn and grow in new ways over time.

Feelings of isolation are common in therapeutic and psychiatric work, particularly in private practice. Preserving confidentiality necessitates that clinicians not talk about clinical work, and the stories they hear daily are often emotionally intense. For mental health professionals, having an ongoing outlet to discuss difficult cases and reflect on how work is variably feeding or draining them is essential. In private practice, proactively building support structures requires greater intentionality and is even more essential because there are limited opportunities for the type of incidental support that can occur in systems where colleagues are in the next office or meet regularly for agency business. The pressure to see a certain number of patients to maintain a steady revenue stream can deter psychiatrists and psychologists from building more professional social support in the form of business lunches, attending talks, or seeking consultation. However, considering consultation, whether formal or informal, is a necessary investment in one's business.

Increasingly, training programs are recognizing the benefits of peer support systems, including the formal mentoring of more junior students by senior individuals in medical school, residency, and doctoral programs, as well as process groups focusing on mindfulness, self-reflection, and open sharing of common experiences. More than a dozen universities (e.g., Vanderbilt, Stanford, Yale, University of Michigan) have published descriptions of their physician wellness programs for medical students and/or medical residents in keeping with the American Medical Association's promotion of such frameworks. Several of these programs have documented promising preliminary findings demonstrating feasibility; satisfaction; and reductions in resident trainee exhaustion, stress, and anxiety (Baker and Sen 2016). These programs variably offer peer advocacy, process groups, meditation-based practice trainings, and faculty-provided psychotherapy tailored to pragmatic trainee concerns (e.g., intake evaluations that are not documented in the medical record; on-site, after-hours appointments to better accommodate rigorous schedules).

Culture of Living Well

Whereas therapy was once viewed from a deficit model that emphasizes diagnosis and treatment of illness, symptom reduction, and management of psychopathology, there is an increasing push in the field toward models of well-being with emphasis on preventive medicine, ongoing self-care, life span practice, and promotion of inspired living. As the field has increasingly embraced third-wave psychotherapies, which emphasize mindfulness, acceptance, and self-compassion, the time is ripe for a cultural change regarding mental health treatment needed by mental health professionals. This new mind-set includes creating training cultures that emphasize the humanity of the clinician and the importance of caring for oneself, including via personal practices, psychotherapy, and psychopharmacology when relevant. Many physician wellness programs invite individuals in leadership to speak about personal struggles and engagement with treatment (Chaukos et al. 2018).

The following case example illustrates how work and personal responsibilities can accumulate to such a point that physical and mental well-being suffer. In addition, the example reveals the pressure mental health professionals can feel to hide anything that can be perceived as a weakness and to appear "fine" in front of colleagues and trainees.

Case Example

Stella Randolph, a mid-career academic psychiatrist, has a reputation within her department and the community as an exceptional physician. She maintains an active research program with a successful grant record, runs a clinic in her area of expertise, teaches undergraduate courses, advises medical students, volunteers for committees, and always has time to consult with colleagues. Dr. Randolph was promoted early at her university and quickly advanced through the ranks. Often the first in at work and the last to leave, Dr. Randolph is respected for her strong work ethic and praised by junior and senior colleagues alike, as well as her trainees and her patients, all of whom regularly comment that they "don't know how she does it all." Dr. Randolph herself does not know how she "does it all" and, in fact, has a niggling feeling that her current pace may not be sustainable. This concern is exacerbated by her increasing difficulty with falling asleep and a recent spike in cluster headaches. However, she is too busy to stop and reflect.

With an upcoming grant deadline, her committee work, and the mounting letters of recommendations for her trainees, Dr. Randolph has no room to slow down and take stock. At her annual medical screening for her university's employee health program, she learns her blood pressure is elevated to an unhealthy level. The nurse completing her screening inquires about lifestyle changes. Dr. Randolph looks pained, and after a sigh, she says she might get up even earlier in the morning to complete workouts before she leaves for the office. The nurse gently wonders if Dr. Randolph might be ignoring the root of the problem by adding one more "to-do" to her already packed and demanding schedule. She encourages Dr. Randolph to make an appointment with a therapist to talk about how she might engage in self-care in a way that is supportive of herself. Dr. Randolph experiences a rush of relief at the idea but quickly dismisses it. She is the one her colleagues come to for support and advice, the one who models how women can "have it all" and break barriers in the workplace. How would it be viewed if she were to start seeing a therapist?

This scenario speaks to the culture of overdoing, the myth of the invulnerable provider, and the stigma associated with seeking treatment. It also highlights that mental health professionals do not need to have clinical levels of symptoms to benefit from formal support. Insomnia, headaches, and feelings of being overwhelmed can be early warning signs that could lead to burnout if not proactively addressed. As a respected faculty physician, Dr. Randolph has an opportunity to contribute to a more positive wellness culture in the field. By openly seeking an outlet to discuss how to balance and integrate self-care in her life, she would be modeling healthy limits and normalizing therapy as a self-care tool for her colleagues and trainees.

Positive Practices

1. Build a consultation group. Trainees in their final years of formal education can often feel saturated by supervision, eager to be licensed and free to practice on their own. Once they are done with formal education, psychiatrists and psychologists typically are reminded of just how valuable this outlet is for their well-being and for optimization of patient care. Formal consultation is no longer as plentiful or free. Every practicing clinician should have a mechanism for receiving consultation and mentorship. In assessing needs, consider the following:

   - **Formality:** Am I seeking formal consultation, such as the consistency of a weekly group, or to increase the frequency with which I access informal consultation (e.g., chatting with a colleague about a specific case on occasion)?
   - **Expertise and facilitation:** Am I looking to enhance specific skills or learn a new technique that might benefit from a paid consultant, or would a peer-led group of respected colleagues be sufficient?
   - **Length:** Is the situation a one-time issue (e.g., needing an ethics or legal consult), or am I seeking a place for ongoing feedback and support?
   - **Content:** Is my desired area of growth focused on a common theme such as a particular treatment approach (e.g., cognitive-behavioral therapy, acceptance and commitment therapy), specialty area (e.g., eating disorders, trauma), or other theme (e.g., building a private practice)?
   - **Participants:** Consider whether your group would comprise people who already work together, those who know each other through less regular contact such as conferences, or a completely open group.
   - **Setting:** Consider the pros and cons of joining an existing group (ease) versus building one (potentially with a more tailored fit) and whether it will be exclusively in-person versus remote, capitalizing on telecommunication.

2. Take a week to intentionally listen to and observe how others in your field talk (or do not communicate) about their own use of mentorship, consultation, therapy, and pharmacotherapy. Are the topics an open part of conversation? Are these practices viewed with respect or judgment? Are some types of support seen as more acceptable than

others? Consider sharing what you are learning about clinician wellness. Ask colleagues about their views of mental health care for the mental health professional and experiences of stigma. If this practice is already comfortable and easy for you, look for ways that you can model openness about seeking care, sharing with mentees when relevant about your own self-care practices, including sharing if you have mentors or a formal consultant or have sought therapy yourself and how it has enhanced your professional and personal well-being.

3. Practice getting the most from therapy, formal consultation, or informal peer-to-peer discussions. As mental health professionals, we are not immune to the desire to be the "good patient" or to be liked by doctors. In fact, some evidence suggests that this problem is exacerbated when health professionals are patients. Say, instead, what is toughest for you right now in your work or your life. Share the doubts or thoughts about yourself or your work that you normally never share. Use your self-knowledge to your advantage by "calling yourself out." Tell your clinician the ways that you typically avoid answering questions, the topics you skirt, or signs you are not sharing as fully or deeply as you might so that your therapist can help you to take full advantage of treatment. State outright any urges you have to not burden your therapist, to appear as a competent professional, or to otherwise behave as a model patient so that you can discuss them. Commit to letting your health professional see every aspect of yourself.

Conclusion

Clinicians deserve the benefits of mental health care as much as their patients do. Whether through ongoing psychotherapy, a contemplative practice, clinical consultation, or peer support, psychiatrists and psychologists would do well to seek support across the course of their careers. The benefits of clinician wellness are exponential because seeking psychotherapy enhances the well-being of both the clinician and the clinician's entire caseload of patients. Specific needs change across the life span and clinical practice, and mental health professionals are fortunate to live in a time when technology and an evolving wellness lens make consultation with and treatment by experts widely accessible. Seeking psychotherapy is not an admission of impairment but an act of commitment to the self and the profession. Embrace the opportunity to experience a different treatment approach, learn a new aspect of the profession, enjoy the support of a weekly meeting, and promote the practice of self-care for future generations of mental health professionals.

Exercise

────────o────────

Confront your core beliefs. Mental health professionals are aware of social and cognitive processing biases. They know that people often give automatic or socially acceptable answers to questions that allow them to maintain an internal sense of consistency between values and actions and that doing so can block awareness of core beliefs and primary emotions. With this in mind, try to answer the following questions for yourself with your heart of hearts, making contact with what is true at your core, even if it makes no sense to your mind or you notice judgment arises. If it makes you squirm, you are doing it "right"!

Have you ever sought psychotherapy? If so, when and for what?

If your answer was yes—

How did you decide that it was time to seek treatment?

_____

_____

_____

How would you know if it was a good time for you to seek treatment again?

_____

_____

_____

What did you gain from seeking psychotherapy? What might you want to gain if you were to seek therapy again, now or in the future?

_____

_____

_____

If your experience was a good one, what made it positive for you? If it was negative, what did not work about the experience? Do you know how to make it positive in the future? If not, how might you seek ideas about improving the experience?

_____

_____

_____

If your answer was no—

Why have you never sought therapy?

_____

_____

_____

What are your beliefs about the function of therapy in people's lives and what it says about them if they seek it?

_____

_____

_____

Are these beliefs the same for yourself as they are for others?

_____

_____

_____

Under which conditions would you seek therapy?

_____

_____

_____

If you decide to seek therapy, would you know how to find a good therapist fit and navigate potential dual relationships comfortably?

_____

_____

_____

———————O———————

Recommended Resources

Baker K, Sen S: Healing medicine's future: prioritizing physician trainee mental health. AMA J Ethics 18(6):604–613, 2016

Geller JD, Norcross JC, Orlinsky DE (eds): The Psychotherapist's Own Psychotherapy: Patient and Clinician Perspectives. New York, Oxford University Press, 2005

Myers MF, Gabbard GO: The Physician as Patient: A Clinical Handbook for Mental Health Professionals. Washington, DC, American Psychiatric Publishing, 2009

Norcross JC, Strausser DJ, Faltus FJ: The therapist's therapist. Am J Psychotherapy 42(1): 53–66, 1988

References

Baker K, Sen S: Healing medicine's future: prioritizing physician trainee mental health. AMA J Ethics 18(6):604–613, 2016 27322994

Barnett JE, Hillard D: Psychologist distress and impairment: the availability, nature, and use of colleague assistance programs for psychologists. Prof Psychol Res Pr 32(2):205–210, 2001

Barnett JE, Baker EK, Elman NS, Schoener GR: In pursuit of wellness: the self-care imperative. Prof Psychol Res Pr 38(6):603–612, 2007

Bennett-Levy J, Finlay-Jones A: The role of personal practice in therapist skill development: a model to guide therapists, educators, supervisors and researchers. Cogn Behav Ther 47(3):185–205, 2018 29485313

Brimstone R, Thistlewaite JE, Quirk F: Behaviour of medical students in seeking mental and physical health care: exploration and comparison with psychology students. Med Educ 14(1), 74–83, 2007 17209895

Chaukos D, Vestal HS, Bernstein CA, et al: An ounce of prevention: a public health approach to improving physician well-being. Acad Psychiatry 42(1):150–154, 2018 28685352

Houpy JC, Lee WW, Woodruff JN, Pincavage AT: Medical student resilience and stressful clinical events during clinical training. Med Educ Online 22(1):1320187, 2017 28460570

Mahoney MJ: Psychotherapists' personal problems and self-care patterns. Prof Psychol Res Pr 28(1):14–16, 1997

Moutier C, Cornette M, Lehrmann J, et al: When residents need health care: stigma of the patient role. Acad Psychiatry 33(6):431–441, 2009 19933883

Norcross JC: The psychotherapist's own psychotherapy: educating and developing psychologists. Am Psychol 60(8):840–850, 2005 16351423

Orlinsky DE, Rønnestad MH: How Psychotherapists Develop: A Study of Therapeutic Work and Professional Growth. Washington, DC, American Psychological Association, 2005

Orlinsky DE, Norcross JC, Rønnestad MH, Wiseman H: Outcomes and impacts of the psychotherapist's own psychotherapy: a research review, in The Psychotherapist's Own Psychotherapy: Patient and Clinician Perspectives. Edited by Geller JD, Norcross JC, Orlinsky DE. New York, Oxford University Press, 2005, pp 214–230

Thomas SJ, Caputi P, Wilson CJ: Specific attitudes which predict psychology students' intentions to seek help for psychological distress. J Clin Psychol 70(3):273–282, 2014 23818259

CHAPTER 14

Meaningful Professional Contributions

Far and away the best prize that life has to offer is the chance to work hard at work worth doing.

Theodore Roosevelt

Psychiatry, psychology, and the related mental health fields are some of the most meaningful and rewarding professions imaginable. When mental health care professionals are effective, they help alleviate the suffering of patients and enhance life satisfaction and well-being. This important mission is the primary reason why clinicians are inspired to enter the mental health field. Providing mental health care can be deeply meaningful and a source of professional and personal fulfillment. Innovative contributions to mental health research, education, and practice have the potential for significant impact on the well-being of future generations.

One of the great paradoxes in the study of burnout is that similar sets of circumstances can contribute to highly variable professional outcomes. An individual's sense that his or her professional contribution is valued is a key driver of professional well-being. The opportunity to pursue meaningful work and receive recognition, involvement in leadership activities and professional development, and effective regulatory and business practices all contribute to the mental health of employees. How well an individual's professional aspirations, personal values, and strengths match the nature of his or her work also has tremendous impact on personal fulfillment. When clinicians are able to make meaning-ful professional contributions, the benefits can be great, not just for the clinician's own wellness but for society at large. In this chapter, we focus on these important issues and review both the challenges and potential benefits of finding meaning in work.

High-Impact Work

The mental health profession can be a compelling career choice. Fore-most, such a career can provide opportunities to make a significant posi-tive impact in the lives of patients. The nature of the work is complex and requires creativity. As a discipline embracing science and existential ques-tions, there is room for curiosity and personal growth. When choosing a career in mental health care, the health professional chooses a career with potential for meaning, challenge, camaraderie, personal growth, and soci-etal impact (Roberts 2013). When clinicians have a strong sense of mean-ing in their work, this may contribute to professional vitality and buffer against feelings of burnout (Seritan 2013).

Perceived lack of personal accomplishment is a core component of the burnout triad of symptoms. Physicians with symptoms of burnout are less likely to find their work rewarding or think their work makes the world a better place. In a study of primary care physicians and psychia-trists in the United States, Jager and colleagues (2017) reported that 42% of respondents strongly agreed that their practice of medicine was a call-ing. As shown in Figure 14–1, a high sense of work as a calling is associated with lower burnout. When working in the field of medicine is no longer personally rewarding, physician performance and patient quality of care are likely to decline.

Professional Effectiveness and Work Satisfaction

Professional effectiveness, defined as the ability to accomplish meaningful work, is directly related to work satisfaction. A healthy professional en-vironment should have room for efficient work that is also personally satisfying to employees. In most workplaces, achieving a healthy work-place requires a balance between personal autonomy, teamwork, and supportive leadership (Alameddine et al. 2009). When work is perceived as especially challenging or frustrating, emotional exhaustion is not al-ways the end result. Long hours, fatigue, and personal sacrifices may be much more tolerable when they are the result of deep focus on a project

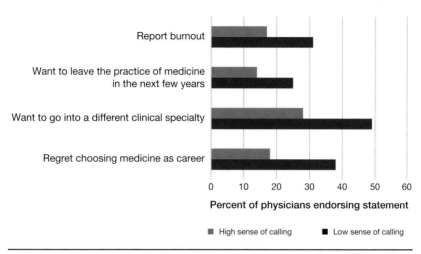

FIGURE 14–1. Sense of calling in relation to physician burnout.

Source. Adapted from Jager et al. 2017.

of personal interest or professional meaning (Moutier 2013). Working hard on an important mission can be inspiring and bring great personal and professional fulfillment.

Extensive literature has covered job engagement and the importance of psychological empowerment in the workplace. According to one theory of organizational empowerment, an employee's sense of empowerment determines an individual's level of motivation to work and, consequently, a wide range of work attitudes and behaviors (Fan et al. 2016). The extent of empowerment in this model depends on several important factors, including support from colleagues at multiple levels across the organization; access to material, financial, and/or human resources; information about organizational decisions; and goals and opportunities for professional growth. When professionals feel as if their efforts have minimal effect, burnout often results. Feeling hopeless—that nothing one does matters in the big picture—can make a professional feel tempted to quit trying.

In several studies of nurses, for example, psychological empowerment was found to be a direct contributor to job engagement. Nurses reporting greater empowerment at work also reported greater fulfillment and higher levels of vigor, dedication, and absorption—the very factors known to directly protect against burnout (Spence Laschinger et al. 2009). Alignment between institutional goals and personal values is important for job engagement as well. When professionals feel that their own vision is not well aligned with the institution's vision, this is a major contributor to job dissatisfaction and even departure from the field. Specifically, feelings of empowerment have been associated with nurses' career satisfaction (Spence Laschinger 2012) and alignment between organizational and clinician values (Vinje and Mittlemark 2008). Psychological safety and the feeling that work and input are valued are key drivers of professional fulfillment and lower rates of burnout.

Types of Contributions

Mental health professionals can make meaningful contributions to both the field and the greater good of society. Some professionals will choose to dedicate themselves primarily to clinical practice and the noble goal of providing high-quality care, one patient at a time. Others will spend time in educational activities and focus their efforts on teaching and training the next generation. Some professionals will prioritize their commitment to advancing the science of mental health care and dedicate time to developing and implementing research projects designed to answer critical questions about the nature of mental illness or the development of effective treatments. Still others will focus energy on disseminating knowledge by publishing academic texts or more general materials for public consumption, or they will work as advocates to influence policy or business practices affecting individuals with mental illness. Regardless of one's role, a growing body of research suggests that generosity in interactions with others is often vital to professional success (Grant 2014).

The type of contribution that is most meaningful may also vary depending on one's career stage. Trainees will likely have many meaningful experiences of clinical care and of discovering new resources and treatment techniques. Early-career individuals often find that teaching others what they have learned is a powerful way to consolidate expertise and feel as if they are making an impact. Later in one's career, mentoring can bring professional satisfaction, or advocacy for policy changes within an organization or local government can seem most rewarding. As individuals approach retirement, it may be important to invest time in making sure that the programs they created and led will continue after they leave the workforce. Many older professionals find great satisfaction from reviewing the professional legacy, whether large or small, that they leave behind when retiring.

Whether you are just beginning your professional career or looking to enhance professional contributions after working for some time, it can be helpful to ask how well aspirations, personal values, and strengths match the nature of the work you are doing. For instance, ask, "What part of being a psychiatrist or psychologist do I find most meaningful?" and "What aspects of my work do I find most motivating?" If you find yourself without much sense of meaning in your current work, think back to a time when there was a feeling of a greater sense of purpose. Perhaps there are aspects of that prior work that you can incorporate now. Table 14–1 outlines key factors observed in professionals who have made major and meaningful professional contributions (Roberts and Hilty 2017).

It is also important to consider to what extent your personal strengths align with the goals of the institution where you are working. Career success is often a matter of good fit between personal values and institutional priorities (Girod 2013). It may take time to figure out what you feel most passionate about, but once you know, make sure that you are able to work within an organization that also has similar values.

A Sense of Meaning in Work

Regardless of the type of work actually done on a daily basis, a sense of connection between work and a higher purpose may be one of the most important contributors to job satisfaction. Across professions, individuals who regard their work as meaningful report greater happiness. This is true even for jobs where the connection with higher meaning is less clear, such as in manufacturing and janitorial services (Coleman 2017).

Although it may be easier to connect some aspects of work, such as teaching, clinical care, or research, with a sense of commitment to the greater good, many necessary tasks in each person's work life can feel tiresome or pointless. Consider parts of the job that feel like busywork. Is there a way to connect these tasks with an important value or mission? Read over the examples in Table 14–2 and look for one that is relatable.

Acknowledgment of Contributions

Although the individual's own sense of meaningful work is critical, public acknowledgment of his or her contributions can also give a significant boost to the sense of professional fulfillment (Menon and Trockel 2019). When a professional is directly thanked by a colleague or supervisor for completing an important task, this show of appreciation can combat the low sense of achievement considered to be a key contributor to burnout (Moutier 2013). Acknowledgment is a core need, and many institutions have formalized processes for recognizing employees, whether through

---

TABLE 14–1. Key qualities in individuals making meaningful
professional contributions

---

1. Sense of purpose
2. Willingness to engage in hard work
3. Commitment to self-care and self-sustenance
4. Creativity
5. Being organized
6. Tenacity and resilience
7. Ability to build a reservoir of good will
8. Insight, intuition, and openness to opportunity

Source. Reprinted from Roberts LW, Hilty DM: "Approaching Your Academic Career," in *Handbook of Career Development in Academic Psychiatry and Behavioral Sciences.* Edited by Roberts LW, Hilty DM. Washington, DC, American Psychiatric Association Publishing, 2017, p. 4. Copyright © 2017 American Psychiatric Association. Used with permission.

an employee-of-the-month program or other types of awards or certificates of achievement. Relatively simple tasks, such as including accolades in agency newsletters, posting accomplishments on a bulletin board, or giving credit for a job well done during a team meeting, can create a culture of appreciation.

Consider your workplace and the extent to which the culture is one of appreciation and acknowledgment for good work. Could credit be given publicly to a colleague for helping with a particular project? How do colleagues typically share information about each other's accomplishments? Are there other programs or actions that could be done to make the good work of others more visible within the organization?

Choosing Meaning

The more clarity there is about the aspects of work that are personally meaningful, the easier it is to take action to follow these passions and make sure meaningful professional contribution is a key part of one's work life. Practical considerations such as schedule, location, pay, and benefits, as well as professional considerations such as the nature of daily work, contacts with colleagues, and opportunities for advancement, all contribute significantly to decision-making about whether a job is a good fit for a particular professional. Ultimately, however, alignment between personal values and institutional mission can have tremendous impact on an individual's long-term work satisfaction. The

TABLE 14–2. Connecting work with meaning

Work task	Connection to meaningful outcome
Timely documentation	Enhances patient safety as an essential component of high-quality care
Covering for a colleague on vacation	Keeps a culture of self-care alive in your agency
Giving difficult feedback to a struggling trainee	Helps a new generation of professionals get ready to do important work in the field
Responding quickly and with compassion to a patient complaint	Fosters the culture of excellence you are proud to be part of
Responsible management of finances	Helps your clinic serve more patients who are unable to pay

following vignettes illustrate how two different professionals made important pivots toward a greater sense of meaning in work.

Vignette

Marie Gillian had been in private practice with psychologist colleagues for 10 years. Although she enjoyed having a high level of control over work-related decision-making and the flexibility to set her own schedule, she felt as if her work was not as impactful and rewarding as she had envisioned when she first began studying psychology. For instance, although she had been able to help patients with anxiety symptoms, she felt frustrated that she could help only one patient at a time.

Over lunch with a colleague, Dr. Gillian confided how she wished she could take the lessons learned from a decade of clinical practice and make them more widely available to people not in therapy. Her colleague suggested creating a professional blog. Itching to work on something new, Dr. Gillian decided to follow through. She scheduled 1 hour per week for writing and soon had enough content for several posts. The more she wrote, the more confident Dr. Gillian felt that she had a worthwhile perspective to share. Her online following grew considerably, and she made many professional connections with peers who had similar interests. The positive feedback encouraged her to reach out to several local companies about presenting lunchtime talks for employees about managing anxiety, her area of expertise. By adding a creative writing outlet for her ideas and giving talks to interested local groups, Dr. Gillian felt she was making a bigger difference for good, the way she had intended to do so many years ago.

Vignette

After completing his psychiatry residency, Bill Fox agreed to take a position within a growing group practice that a few of his friends had joined the year before. He found many aspects of the job attractive, including a brand-new office space, decent salary, and proximity to his home. There was high enough demand for psychiatric care in his local community that he did not need to advertise his services much and soon had a full caseload of patients, in spite of the fact that the office did not accept most medical insurances and many patients paid out of pocket for care. After a year of working, Dr. Fox wished he could help more people who could not afford to pay the high price of visiting the clinic. He thought about how he had been inspired to enter psychiatry when he volunteered at a homeless shelter as a teenager and saw the devastating effects mental illness can have on a person's life. Dr. Fox realized that giving back to his community was a core personal value and essential to feeling fulfilled by his work. He started volunteering at a community clinic on the weekends to provide treatment for underserved populations. He noticed that he felt more inspired by the people he met there and the challenge of the work. When a position was posted for medical director of the community clinic, he decided to apply. When the job was offered to him, it was a hard choice, but the more Dr. Fox reflected on the reasons he had decided to become a psychiatrist, the more he knew he would be happier in a position where he was working with an underserved patient population.

Mentorship

To accomplish meaningful professional contribution, most professionals need mentorship or coaching (Becker and Yager 2013; Van Emmerik 2004). This input may be important at different times during one's career trajectory, both in the early stages of choosing which path to pursue and at later stages as leadership and influence increase. Mentorship can also help with diverse aspects of career development, including enhancing clinical skills, teaching, research, community engagement, or administrative and leadership roles.

Given the diverse roles mentors can play, many professionals need several types of mentors. As discussed in Chapter 2, "Professional and Personal Developmental Milestones," technical mentorships can be short-term relationships with professionals who have specific skills. This type of mentorship is more circumscribed, focused primarily on the development of a particular skill set. These mentors can even work in areas quite different from that of the person being mentored, as long as they possess knowledge relevant to the individual's role. Many different types of technical mentors may also be needed over the course of a psychiatrist's or psychologist's career. If there is a specific skill an individual wants to acquire, looking for a short-term mentoring relationship to provide inspiration and guidance may be quite productive.

Many professionals also benefit from a developmental mentor who serves as a champion for overall career development. These types of mentoring relationships can take longer to develop because they rely on both professional and personal compatibility. If additional mentorship is needed, Becker and Yager (2013) suggest starting with a self-assessment process to determine the type of mentorship desired and the skills the individual brings to the relationship. The more clarity the individual has about his or her mentorship needs, the more easily he or she will be able to identify potential mentoring relationships and establish clear communication at the outset.

Some institutions have formal mentoring programs, which can be a promising way to start. If there is no formal program available, rely on existing professional relationships to identify more senior colleagues who may be open to mentoring and who may share professional interests. Often, working on a collaborative project can be a good way to get started and test the mentoring relationship. Make sure to look not just for individuals with expertise that is valued but also people who are genuinely interested in mentoring.

Another promising area for future research is the development of effective systems within workplaces to formalize mentorship and give professionals access to leadership development activities and executive coaching. Large organizations are recognizing the need to provide leadership training to their executive staff (Shanafelt and Noseworthy 2017). If made more widely available, reasonably priced, and discipline specific, professional development coaching could help mental health professionals enhance their professional impact and personal sense of fulfillment.

Positive Practices

1. There is probably one aspect of your work that you find most personally meaningful. Make sure you spend at least 1 day weekly or at least 1 hour daily focused on a part of your job that is meaningful to you. If this is not possible now, what changes could you make in the future to engage more consistently in meaningful work?
2. Pick a simple action you do every day, such as walking out to the clinic waiting room, unlocking your office door, or entering your computer password, and use this as a daily opportunity to return to a mindful state and reflect on the positive impact you can have be-

fore engaging in work for the day. For example, one doctor used the moment of hand washing before entering a patient's room as an opportunity to do a quick breathing exercise focused on returning to a mindful state just prior to greeting each new family. The practice can help remind you of the meaning in even the simplest of tasks.

3. Sharing what you know is a great way to have a larger impact in your field and make meaningful contributions for colleagues and patients. You have experience and expertise that are valuable. Try to dedicate 15 minutes daily to writing about your area of interest. Even 15 minutes of writing, done consistently, will accumulate into a substantial amount of content over just a few months (Belcher 2009). Write in any format that feels right. Fairly soon, you may find that you have accumulated enough content that you can share more formally on a website or blog post, in an editorial, or even as a formal journal article.

Conclusion

A professional's sense that his or her work is meaningful buffers against burnout and enhances engagement and fulfillment. Mental health care is a challenging profession that also has great inherent potential for meaning. Many aspects of this work can be emotionally exhausting. But when systems support efficient practice, good work is acknowledged, and mentorship for career development is accessible, clinicians across the professional life span can flourish. The extent to which an individual can mentally connect daily tasks with outcomes he or she cares about will likely enhance a sense of engagement and job satisfaction. Over the long term, the extent to which psychiatrists and psychologists can pivot toward working on projects that are personally meaningful will have great influence on professional and personal fulfillment. Best wishes on this important journey!

Exercises

———————o———————

1. **Write down three reasons you were inspired to enter the mental health field.**

_____

_____

_____

2. List which aspects of your personality make you effective
   at your job.

   _____

   _____

   _____

3. List any characteristics that make you vulnerable to compromising self-care.

   _____

   _____

   _____

4. **Write down major categories of professional activities.** In
   a given week, you may be involved in a wide variety of clinical, teaching, research, community engagement, and leadership activities as part of your professional role.

   How personally meaningful are those roles to you? Enter
   a score for each (1=most and 5=least meaningful).

Activity or role	Score

   Now go back and consider which of these missions you
   find most personally meaningful or fulfilling. Write a number in the column on the right reflecting your own rank order

of the activities in terms of personal meaningfulness. Do you engage in work related to your top-ranked activities on a daily or at least weekly basis? If not, take time to adjust your schedule so that each week includes time for the activity that gives you the strongest sense of meaning.

5. **Choose a daily work task to accomplish mindfully**. Pause briefly to reflect on the meaning in your work.

   Write your idea for a daily activity.

   _____

   _____

   _____

   What cues in the environment can you use to remind yourself to be mindful?

   _____

   _____

   _____

6. **Make time to write.** Writing consolidates an individual's thinking and can be a powerful tool for sharing important ideas with others.

   When could you schedule a 15-minute writing block into your day?

   _____

   _____

   _____

What topic of personal interest could you start writing about?

_____

_____

_____

————————o————————

Recommended Resources

Farmer P: Partner to the Poor: A Paul Farmer Reader, Vol 23. Berkeley, University of California Press, 2010

Gawande A: Complications: A Surgeon's Notes on an Imperfect Science. New York, Picador, 2010

Grant A: WorkLife With Adam Grant (podcast audio), 2019. Available at: www.ted.com/podcasts/worklife. Accessed May 31, 2019.

Schulte B: Your Work May Be Killing You (Better Life Lab podcast audio). Washington, DC, New America, 2018. Available at: https://www.newamerica.org/better-life-lab/podcasts/better-life-lab-podcast-your-work-may-be-killing-you/. Accessed March 5, 2019.

References

Alameddine M, Dainty KN, Deber R, Sibbald WJ: The intensive care unit work environment: current challenges and recommendations for the future. J Crit Care 24(2):243–248, 2009 19327295

Becker A, Yager J: How to approach mentorship as a mentee, in The Academic Medicine Handbook: A Guide to Achievement and Fulfillment for Academic Faculty. Edited by Roberts LW. New York, Springer, 2013, pp 157–162

Belcher WL: Writing Your Journal Article in Twelve Weeks: A Guide to Academic Publishing Success. Thousand Oaks, CA, Sage, 2009

Coleman J: To find meaning in your work, change how you think about it. Harvard Business Review, December 29, 2017. Available at https://hbr.org/2017/12/to-find-meaning-in-your-work-change-how-you-think-about-it. Accessed January 5, 2020.

Fan Y, Zheng Q, Liu S, Li Q: Construction of a new model of job engagement, psychological empowerment and perceived work environment among Chinese registered nurses at four large university hospitals: implications for nurse managers seeking to enhance nursing retention and quality of care. J Nurs Manag 24(5):646–655, 2016 27039839

Girod SC: How to align individual goals with institutional goals, in The Academic Medicine Handbook: A Guide to Achievement and Fulfillment for Academic Faculty. Edited by Roberts LW. New York, Springer, 2013, pp 27–31

Grant A: Give and Take: Why Helping Others Drives Our Success. New York, Penguin, 2014

Jager AJ, Tutty MA, Kao AC: Association between physician burnout and identification with medicine as a calling. Mayo Clin Proc 92(3):415–422, 2017 28189341

Menon NK, Trockel MT: Creating a culture of wellness, in The Art and Science of Physician Wellbeing: A Handbook for Physicians and Trainees. Edited by Roberts LW, Trockel MT. Cham, Switzerland, Springer, 2019, pp 19–32

Moutier C: How to have a healthy life balance as an academic physician, in The Academic Medicine Handbook: A Guide to Achievement and Fulfillment for Academic Faculty. Edited by Roberts LW. New York, Springer, 2013, pp 429–435

Roberts LW (ed): The Academic Medicine Handbook: A Guide to Achievement and Fulfillment for Academic Faculty. New York, Springer, 2013

Roberts LW, Hilty DM: Approaching your academic career, in Handbook of Career Development in Academic Psychiatry and Behavioral Sciences. Edited by Roberts LW, Hilty DM. Arlington, VA, American Psychiatric Association Publishing, 2017, pp 3–11

Seritan AL: How to recognize and avoid burnout, in The Academic Medicine Handbook: A Guide to Achievement and Fulfillment for Academic Faculty. Edited by Roberts LW. New York, Springer, 2013, pp 447–453

Shanafelt TD, Noseworthy JH: Executive leadership and physician well-being: nine organizational strategies to promote engagement and reduce burnout. Mayo Clin Proc 92(1):129–146, 2017 27871627

Spence Laschinger HK: Job and career satisfaction and turnover intentions of newly graduated nurses. J Nurs Manag 20(4):472–484, 2012 22591149

Spence Laschinger HK, Wilk P, Cho J, Greco P: Empowerment, engagement and perceived effectiveness in nursing work environments: does experience matter? J Nurs Manag 17(5):636–646, 2009 19575722

Van Emmerik H: For better and for worse: adverse working conditions and the beneficial effects of mentoring. Career Dev Int 9(4):358–373, 2004

Vinje HF, Mittelmark MB: Community nurses who thrive: the critical role of job engagement in the face of adversity. J Nurses Staff Dev 24(5):195–202, 2008 18838896

Index

Page numbers printed in **boldface** type refer to tables and figures.